HERE'S WHAT PEOPLE ARE SAYING ABOUT *ORAL ROBERTS ON HEALING*...

I'd like to introduce you to a man who was called to a generation of people, whom I knew very well, and that was Oral Roberts. I called him Chancellor Roberts. His experiences were phenomenal, his faith was exceptional, but above all, he was what he said. He lived what he said, and he gave people vision at a time when many in the church didn't have a vision. He understood things that many ministers did not understand, and he stepped out by faith to do what God called him to do.

I believe this book will challenge you to believe the unbelievable and receive the impossible because it's doable! What a blessing of the Lord that God chose this wonderful man to preach on healing and to give such revelation that the world so desperately needed to know. He had a lot of persecution, but he had way more miracles than he ever had persecution. I pray this book will change your mind about healing, and you'll know beyond a shadow of doubt that healing IS for today! As you read this book, you will travel through time. You will come to know the man, Oral Roberts, and his mission. But what you will really come to know is the will of God for your life. So let the journey begin!

—*Dr. Jesse Duplantis*
Evangelist, author, TV host
President and founder, Jesse Duplantis Ministries

D1551396

I am grateful Richard Roberts has decided to share his dad's thoughts and experiences in this book. One of the most meaningful and special days in my more-than-sixty-year ministry journey was a meeting I had with Oral. I called and asked if I could meet him privately, and I could tell he was surprised that a conservative Bible Baptist would be asking to have a private time with him. I told him, "Oral, I come to ask for your forgiveness. For years, I belittled and made fun of you. God has brought me under deep conviction, showing me that much of the church and community has cut you off and forced you to become an island unto yourself. I have personally contributed to that un-Christlike, unloving separation. I hope you will forgive me."

Oral began to weep deeply in the first five minutes of our conversation. He said, "You have no idea what this means to me. I've been cut off by my own church and virtually every denomination. Thank you, James. I'm overwhelmed." I was deeply moved and so grateful. I then told him, "I would like to get other church and denominational leaders to have time to sit down with you and hear your heart and let them feel welcome to share theirs."

We set the meeting, and several hundred church leaders gathered with us. It was one of the most Christ-centered, Holy-Spirit-powered gatherings I've been part of, and it impacted Oral deeply, as well as those who attended. We realized how we foolishly force separation among believers over insignificant differences and outright unkindness and lack of love, to say nothing of the importance of unconditional love, which Christ offers everyone. There isn't one of us who doesn't need to experience that unconditional love, but also, we need to learn how to share it.

Oral and I became friends until he went home to be with the Lord. We talked together often and we prayed about the whole family of God. Those moments were special.

I remember his wife, Evelyn, said to me, "James, you and Betty are wonderful. You know that she affirms you, and many people hear and receive you because of your wife. What a blessing she is to you and all of us." I agreed and told her she was the same for Oral.

I'm grateful for the friendship I enjoyed with Oral. I'm grateful I was able to encourage him, help lighten his load and brighten his days and also bring Christian leaders together with a deeper understanding of the importance of spiritual unity and unconditional love.

God bless you, Richard, and above all, dear God, please bring the church family together. Thank you, Richard, and I'm praying God will use what Oral shared to help lead us to supernatural unity and healing.

—*James Robison*
Founder and president, Life Outreach International,
Fort Worth, TX

As a young girl in the 1970s, I would sit riveted in front of our television to watch Oral Roberts' weekly broadcast. It was during those programs that a love for the healing power of God was planted and stoked in me. Oral Roberts was one of the first to introduce me to this divine flow of God's love.

I had no idea then that God would one day lead me to become a student at Oral Roberts University. It was one of the most treasured seasons of my life, as I got to attend weekly chapel services and sit directly under the ministry of Oral Roberts and Richard Roberts. It was in those chapel services that I witnessed firsthand the healing ministry in operation.

Through Oral Roberts, the first seeds of the healing ministry were planted in me. I received divine impartations that have marked and impacted the flow of the healing ministry in my own life. Through many others just like me, the fruit of Oral Roberts' healing ministry is still a living and moving flow in the earth. Although Oral Roberts no longer lives here on the earth, the truths and revelations he imparted are still alive and blessing people today.

As you feast on *Oral Roberts on Healing*, expect to receive your miracle! As he would say, "Every day, miracles are either coming to you or going past you!" In this book, you will learn how to lay hold of that miracle power that is yours today! For as Oral Roberts often stated, "Something good is going to happen to you!"

—*Nancy Dufresne*
Dufresne Ministries, Murrieta, CA

The words of those who greatly impacted the kingdom of God outlive the life they had on earth. Oral Roberts was one of most influential evangelists to demonstrate the power of God through the healing of the body, soul, and spirit. He would be the first to tell you that it was God who heals, not him. This book contains his teaching and life story compiled by my friends Richard and Lindsay Roberts. Pick up a copy with an intent to receive all that God has for you!

—*Joni Lamb*
Cofounder, Daystar Television Network

Oral Roberts was the trailblazer in the healing ministry that set the world ablaze. Miracles had been talked about since the days of Jesus instructing and showing the disciples. Oral Roberts took the Scriptures literally; he believed that we can do the works of Jesus in His name. His example of big faith and big actions was passed on to his son Richard Roberts. This book teaches all of us that something good is going to happen today.

—*Tim Storey*
Author, speaker, and life coach

ORAL ROBERTS ON HEALING

ORAL ROBERTS

ON

HEALING

LIVING IN
GOD'S MIRACLES

WHITAKER
HOUSE

Unless otherwise indicated, all Scripture quotations are taken from the King James Version of the Holy Bible. Scripture quotations marked (NKJV) are taken from the *New King James Version*, © 1982 by Thomas Nelson, Inc. Used by permission. All rights reserved. Scripture quotations marked (NIV) are taken from the *Holy Bible, New International Version*®, NIV®, © 1973, 1978, 1984, 2011 by Biblica, Inc.® Used by permission of Zondervan. All rights reserved worldwide. www.zondervan.com. The "NIV" and "New International Version" are trademarks registered in the United States Patent and Trademark Office by Biblica, Inc.® Scripture quotations marked (ESV) are taken from *The Holy Bible, English Standard Version*, © 2016, 2001, 2000, 1995 by Crossway Bibles, a division of Good News Publishers. Used by permission. All rights reserved. Boldface type in the Scripture quotations indicates the author's emphasis.

ORAL ROBERTS ON HEALING
Living in God's Miracles

richardroberts.org
Richard Roberts Ministries
P.O. Box 2187
Tulsa, OK 74102-2187

ISBN: 979-8-88769-270-8 | eBook ISBN: 979-8-88769-271-5
Printed in the United States of America
© 2024 by Richard Roberts and Lindsay Roberts

Whitaker House
1030 Hunt Valley Circle
New Kensington, PA 15068
www.whitakerhouse.com

Library of Congress Control Number: 2024941555

1 2 3 4 5 6 7 8 9 10 11 ᴗᴗ 31 30 29 28 27 26 25 24

CONTENTS

PART 3: WHAT TO DO IF YOU NEED HEALING

PART 4: HEALING IS IN GOD'S HANDS

FOREWORD

I personally, with my own eyes and with my own heart, witnessed miracles I have never heard of before or since at the tent meetings with Brother Oral Roberts in 1967. One of these miracles occurred when an elderly woman was carried in on an army cot by her nurse. I touched her on the head and spoke the name of Jesus, but Brother Roberts was standing right behind me, and he shouted, "In the name of Jesus Christ of Nazareth, whom I serve, take your hands off God's property now!" She leaned up and spit that malignant cancer from her stomach. Then, she jumped up and ran with the nurse!

Another mighty miracle from those tent meetings was when a nine-year-old girl who came in strapped to a wheelchair received her full healing! That night, Brother Roberts had instructed the audience to move something by faith to receive their healing, and that little girl could move nothing but her eyes. She began moving her eyes as fast as she could and then jumped up and ran like she was in the Olympics!

I don't have the space to tell of all the wonderful miracles that the Lord did in those tent meetings. But I can tell you that Brother Oral Roberts said to me, "The tent anointing is coming back and when it does, it will *be big time!*" I believe that time is now. Don't just read this book; read it with your Bible in hand. Jesus said in John 14:12–13, "*Verily, verily, I say unto you, He that believeth on me, the works that I do shall he do also; and greater works than these shall he do; because I go unto my Father. And whatsoever ye shall ask in my name, that I will do, that the Father may be glorified in the Son.*" He continues to say in John 14:16, "*And I will pray the Father, and he shall give you another Comforter, that he may abide with you for ever.*" Well, the Comforter is here inside you and me. Brother Oral Roberts isn't the miracle worker. Jesus said it's the Father in me who does the work. It is the same Father and Spirit in you, so go boldly into the world and spread the gospel because the tent anointing is back big time!

God loves you, we love you, and *Jesus is Lord!*

—Kenneth Copeland
Founder, Kenneth Copeland Ministries

INTRODUCTION

My father, Oral Roberts, was convinced that prayer is a mighty instrument of healing in God's hand. Nothing could shake him from this strong belief, and he saw it proven in the lives of the many people he ministered to throughout his lifetime. He saw God touch and heal people who had been told they would surely die, restoring their health and giving them full, abundant lives.

He saw and personally experienced God's supernatural, miracle-working power, but he also believed that God uses doctors and other aspects of healthcare to bring healing. He didn't tell God which method to use; he simply knew that God *does* heal, and he remained thankful for that all of his life.

My father was ahead of his time in certain ways. Long before *the mind-body connection* became popular, he believed that negative thoughts and emotions could be healed and line up with God's Word. He came to believe that in addition to God's miraculous touch, doctors, and other godly things, a person's thoughts about himself or herself could also become some of God's instruments of healing as it lined up with the Bible. The Scripture verse that helped him understand this is Luke 10:27 (NKJV), where Jesus says, "'*You shall love the* LORD *your God with all your heart, with all your soul, with all your strength, and with all your mind,*' *and* '*your neighbor as yourself.*'"

He referred to this verse as *the love commandment* and believed that this verse teaches us the importance of right relationships—with God, with other people, and with ourselves. When we love God, love others, and love ourselves properly, great things can happen. Think about it. When we recognize God as the source of our lives and look to Him alone to meet all our needs through whatever method He chooses, we can come into right relationship with Him. When we deal with our personal thoughts, emotions, and habits in biblical ways, we can be in right relationship with ourselves.

His understanding of Luke 10:27 led my father to coin the term *seed faith*, which simply means to plant a seed (meaning to give something) in the area of life in which you want or need to reap a harvest—such as an answered prayer, a God-given dream fulfilled, or some type of need met—believing that God is able to take a small act of faith, bring a great harvest as a result, and trusting Him to do it. My father practiced and preached the idea of seed faith from the time he began to understand it until the day God called him home to heaven. Understanding the power of planting a seed in faith helped him believe he could minister to seriously ill people and offer them hope for healing—and to see God do miracles for them. Understanding the miracle of seed faith helped him believe he could become the founder of a university, appear regularly on prime-time national television, and minister to people with significant problems—physical illness, addiction, financial troubles, family discord, and other situations that seemed impossible—and see them healed, whole, restored, and set free by the power of God.

The principle of seed faith was integral to my father's ministry, and it's integral to this book. Portions of this book were originally published in 1961. Other portions were published in 1976 and revised in 1981 or published in 1947 and re-released in 2002. In addition, our library archives contain notes and materials up to my father's home-going to heaven in 2009, so we have expanded his original books with many of his personal notes and conversations we had with him. I have also gleaned from personal discussions and close workings with Dad in what I consider to be the most valuable time I had the privilege to spend learning about the Bible over my entire lifetime.

My wife Lindsay had worked closely with my dad on many projects over several decades. With her help and careful preservation of his uniquely insightful ministry materials, I have gathered selected portions of material from these works. This book would not exist without Lindsay's care and diligence. My father called her a daughter as the two of them were extremely close. He trusted her with his writings and materials. I am forever grateful for her dedication, for that of my family, and also for the help of Dr. Jeff Ogle in completing this project.

Because of the continued interest in Oral Roberts and his material, this tells me that his teachings and his message are not limited to a particular time period. We know that people have suffered with sickness, lack, and other struggles for years and that many today—perhaps even you—are searching for hope and solutions to their problems. That's why I am honored to make this book available to you, as it contains some of my father's most important teachings on healing. If you need a miracle today, in your own life or for someone you love, I believe this book is a great place to start.

I've asked my close friend and *New York Times* best-selling author Dr. Don Colbert to share his thoughts on whole-person healing. He was both a student of my father's ministry and one of my father's personal physicians. I pray his insight on this book will be a blessing to you concerning healing, and I pray this book ministers to you in every way possible.

—*Richard Roberts*

A PERSONAL NOTE FROM DON COLBERT

Oral Roberts had a gift in the area of divine health and healing. His gift involved not only praying for people to be healed but also seeing remarkable miracles take place. He also understood and practiced the importance of people taking care of their health and recognized that although God does work miracles, He also wants us to partner with Him concerning our health.

As far as I know, Oral Roberts was the first person to integrate divine healing with taking care of our bodies. He believed the saying, "What you can do, God will not do. But what you cannot do, God will do." He was a pioneer of merging together the natural with the supernatural, a vital combination. Also, he had a powerful impact on my life as a physician, in my spiritual life, and in my personal life.

When I was a student at the Oral Roberts University School of Medicine, one of the requirements for every student was to be a part of an exercise program. This was not optional; it was mandatory. In addition, Oral Roberts taught students the importance of healthy eating combined with exercise. He stressed the importance of taking care of ourselves as *"the temple of the Holy Spirit"* (1 Corinthians 6:19 NKJV) and knew that caring properly for one's physical body helps bring natural healing. Oral Roberts' teaching about taking care of our temple and believing God for miracles has greatly influenced me both personally and professionally in my practice as a medical doctor.

During my time as a student, I suffered a massive heat stroke, a medical incident so severe I almost died. I was told I would lose the use of my legs and never walk again. But I was in an environment filled with prayers and believing God, and it was there that God did a miraculous thing in restoring my health and the use of my legs. I personally received a major miracle while in the atmosphere of prayer and healing. This heightened my ability to believe in miracles and reinforced my belief that what we do in the natural realm to take care of our bodies is important. The influence of what I learned and experienced under Oral Roberts' ministry has been the driving force behind me and my ministry to this day.

I believe that Oral Roberts was one of the greatest teachers of the Bible and life lessons of my time. His teachings were the foundation on which many others and I have received revelation of healing and miracles, and I have carried these truths into my medical practice, implemented them with my patients, and applied them personally. I believe those of us who knew and learned from Oral Roberts have a job to do, which is to help carry his powerful message to those who need hope and healing today. It's important that his message continues today, and that's why I'm delighted to see this book made available to a new generation of people all over the world.

—*Don Colbert, M.D.*

PART 1

GET TO KNOW THE MIRACLE-WORKER

1

MY MIRACULOUS HEALING

As you begin this book, I want to share with you the story of the miraculous physical healing God did in my life when I was a young man. I believe He heals in every way. He heals our bodies. He heals our minds. He heals our emotions. He heals our relationships. He heals our finances. In whatever way we need healing, God is able to bring it to pass for us. He did it for me, and as the apostle Peter said in Acts 10:34, He "*is no respecter of persons.*" What He has done for one person, He can do for another.

I want you to know that I understand what it feels like to need healing. You'll quickly see that I was extremely ill at one time, and God healed me. When I write about healing, I do so with compassion for all who are sick or infirmed in any way and with confidence that God wants to heal us and is our Healer based on Exodus 15:26:

> *If thou wilt diligently hearken to the voice of the LORD thy God, and wilt do that which is right in his sight, and wilt give*

*ear to his commandments, and keep all his statutes, I will put none of these diseases upon thee, which I have brought upon the Egyptians: for **I am the LORD that healeth thee.***

Let me share my testimony of the struggles I faced as a young person and the testimony of God's healing touch in my life, so that as you read this book, you can know that I have firsthand experience with adversities, serious illness, and God's miraculous healing power.

MY CROSS AND MY CROWN

As a child, I was well acquainted with poverty and spent many long hours picking cotton to help out our family. We never had *enough*, and I always knew it. We were so in need that I remember my family saying that even the poor people called us poor. I never fully understood it at the time, but I did know that it wasn't good.

Life seemed to present challenge after challenge. For me, one of the greatest challenges was that I stuttered badly. One of my father's family members thought the world of me, but because he teased me, I thought he hated me. One day after a particularly humiliating experience in which he seemed to encourage a crowd in our home to laugh at my attempt to talk, I slipped away and hid under the house. After they left about sundown, I crawled out and stood on the back porch of the little house where I had been born. Barefoot and dressed in overalls, I looked out across the hills upon Pontotoc County, Oklahoma, and wondered what was on the other side and if I would ever amount to anything. Standing there, I felt lost and hopeless, bewildered, confused, frustrated, and afraid. I saw nothing in myself, and neither did anyone else, except for my siblings and my parents.

Papa had said to this man, "Why don't you let Oral alone? God has His hand on him. Someday he will preach the gospel and then you will be sorry." However, Papa's family member just laughed and said, "Oral, preach? Why, he can't even talk." He thought it was a big joke. But Papa said, "Someday you will see."

Before his death, that relative and I became very close. When I returned to Ada, Oklahoma, for a revival crusade in 1948, he came and accepted Christ as his personal Savior. After that, he sincerely served God and supported my ministry with his prayers.

I was born a stutterer, but God showed Mama the day would come that He would heal me. I was persecuted at school, where the other students tried to get me to talk. The ridicule never seemed to stop. My classmates laughed and eventually the teacher would laugh until finally I would run home in humiliation. There, Mama would somehow know just what to say; she reminded me that someday my tongue would be loosed, and I would preach. I thought I kept that quiet, but Mama's words must've spilled forth in my conversation. Soon, the boys at school tagged me as a preacher. When I came near, they would laugh and say, "There's the preacher. Why don't you preach a sermon?" After those boys chased me home that day, I told my chief tormentor that I would get him someday when I was grown.

Years later in our crusade in Oklahoma City, a nicely dressed man stopped me as I entered in the tent cathedral to preach. He said, "Remember me?" I took one look and started to say, "How could I ever forget you?" but thought the better of it. Yes, it was the main bully from my school days. After greeting him, I went ahead to preach and at the invitation to come to the altar, the first to come forward to make a decision for Christ was my *friend*. After his conversion, I smiled as I realized I had gotten even with him all right, but it was not like I had expected.

When I graduated from grade school, I was elected the king of my class and was to be presented with the queen in the final assembly program at the end of the term. I hurried home and told Papa I needed special clothes so I could look the part of a king. Papa was a preacher who had to depend on the free offerings of the people to whom he ministered. Sometimes we had plenty; sometimes we had nothing. Sometimes it was as though the people believed their preacher should be humble and poor—if God would keep him humble, they would keep him poor.

Papa was unable at that time to buy new clothes for the class *king*, so I got a job selling the *Ada Evening News* after school and bought my own *royal wardrobe*. It wasn't much, but I was proud of it: a new denim shirt, a pair of overalls, and a new pair of tennis shoes. No socks or tie. The whole outfit cost me $2.16. I remember the amount distinctly. But when I walked into the school room in all my glory, the teacher said, "Shouldn't you run home and dress?" I said, "I'm dressed. Put the crown on my head." I had worked hard to buy those clothes, and they looked good to me. The queen was waiting to be escorted into the assembly room. She was the daughter of a rich family and was dressed in white satin. Wearing my two-dollar clothes, I escorted her while the band played. We were crowned and presented. The queen bowed; the king bowed. For once I felt like I was every inch of king.

MOTHER'S PRAYERS FOLLOWED ME

I grew up wanting to become a lawyer. At the age of fifteen, I had my own set of law books in addition to my schoolbooks. I was fascinated by the study of law. Politics also interested me. My secret ambition was to pass the bar examination and later become governor of Oklahoma.

What I did not know, although Mama and Papa knew, was that all this was part of the preparation to follow the plan God had made for me before I was born. The powerful force motivating me today is no stronger than it was when I was a teenage lad with a passion inside to become a lawyer and governor of my state. The difference now is that I know why I feel the passion, and I know where it is leading me.

Mama and Papa did not want me to dabble in politics. They had a terrible fear that it might engulf me and take my interest away from the call they felt I had from God. I remember things they told me about this call from my earliest childhood.

It was hard for them to get me to listen. I was always busy. My mind and hands wanted to be doing something. I didn't want to stop and listen to their talk about religion.

My parents had "religion" in the home as well as in church. Jesus Christ was an integral part of our family life. When I was small, I actually thought He lived at our house. I couldn't see Him as a person, but Mama and Papa talked to Him personally and often. Their keynote message to us children was: "Jesus will take care of you." Each of us five children was raised to accept this as naturally as we breathed. All problems great and small were taken to Jesus.

When my parents learned of my plans to leave home shortly before my sixteenth birthday, they were hurt and begged me not to go. Finally, my mother burst out, "Oral, there is something God wants you to do with your life. This has been made clear to your father and me." Now my mother always had a way of talking to me that reached inside me. It never occurred to me to doubt her. She said, "Son, don't be hard to manage and throw your life away. Don't miss God's calling."

The big difficulty in my mind then was that she spoke too much about Christianity. It was all right for them ... but I had other plans.

I had dreamed of leaving home for months. At my age, I felt I lived in a different world from theirs. Their life revolved around God. I respected them and their faith, but I was not ready for that kind of life. I wanted to live my own life. I felt I could take care of myself. Also, I wanted to *make something of myself*—to get away from a life I considered too narrow and restricted. I wanted to reach the top.

This is not to say that I did not know what Mama was talking about. As a child, there were many times when I felt close to God. Through my parents, I had come to know God and who He was.

Mama touched a tender spot that day before I left. When she saw my determination to leave, it seemed to dawn upon her that I was no longer her baby. I was over six feet tall, and I felt that I was my own person. Still, she almost succeeded in stopping me. "Oral, you go on, but remember this: You will never be able to go beyond our prayers. Each day, we will pray and ask God to send you home." She and Papa asked me to kneel with them and I did. If there is anything to being *branded in prayer*, they branded me in prayer that day. They prayed, "O Lord, this is our baby boy. You gave him to us, and we have given him back to You. He is leaving us to go on his own. Now we commit his young life into Your loving hands. Watch over him and bring him back to us. In Jesus's name. Amen."

After that prayer, I almost backed out of my decision to leave. They had appealed to another side of me that I had known was there and deeply respected. But with the excitement of youth, I had my own way and walked out of their house and their lives. I never intended to return. In the southern part of Oklahoma where I went to live, I secured a job in a judge's home. I had access to his fine library of law books, which I began to study with all the hunger of a young animal searching for food.

FAR FROM HOME—AND GOD

During the year that I was gone, I felt a million miles away from my parents. They sent me many loving letters and ended each one by saying, "Son, don't forget God. Remember, each day, we call your name in prayer." There were times when my mind went back to my childhood, recalling the exciting experiences my brother Vaden and I had in the summertime, traveling with Papa when he held revival meetings.

But except for the few times I felt a *"still small voice"* (1 Kings 19:12) whispering to me, I lived as if I had never known anything at all about God. I was my own boss, kept my own hours, and did what I wanted to do.

I laid out a demanding schedule for myself. Besides going to school, I held down three part-time jobs and completely supported myself. I was a handyman in the judge's home, I worked in a store on Saturdays, and I became a reporter for my hometown paper, the *Ada Evening News*.

My lessons were easy for me; I loved to study, and I was an "A" student. My goal was to make something of myself, and I worked hard at it. I was elected president of my class and made the basketball team.

I paid no attention to the pain that started in my chest or the night sweats upon my bed. I grew tired easily. I was always busy with basketball and expended as much energy on the court as I did anything else I was involved in. Many times, I felt my lungs would explode before I finished a game. By this time, I was spitting up a little blood now and then but thought nothing of it. I was caught up in the fascination of making my own way. Supremely happy in my new life, I felt nothing could stop me or slow me down.

Six months had passed since I had left home. Then seven, then eight. By this time, my mind had become more or less separated from my parents and from what they represented in "religion."

But at age seventeen, my great dream suddenly became a nightmare. Within a period of twenty-four hours, my world crumbled about me. I collapsed on the court while playing in the final game for the Southern Oklahoma District Basketball Championship. While dribbling toward the basket to make a layup shot that would win the game, I felt life going out of my lungs. I fell upon the gymnasium floor, with blood running from my mouth. My coach, Herman Hamilton, rushed over, picked me up, and wrapped me in his topcoat. He leaned over me and said, "Oral, you're going home. I'm taking you today."

Lying in the back seat of Mr. Hamilton's car, I felt my life was shattered. But I knew that the prayers of my godly parents were catching up with me.

MY HEALING MIRACLE

Now, I found myself bedridden with the deadly diagnosis of tuberculosis. In my eagerness to make it on my own, I had ignored all the symptoms. In the 1930s, tuberculosis meant the victim was doomed. There was no medical cure. So when the doctor gave my parents the diagnosis, it was a death sentence, and it shook our family. The days and nights that stretched out before us were terribly dark. Many nights, I saw my mother and father on bended knee, asking God to save me and heal my body. The doctors continued to say that there was no hope left for me.

My physical body began to decline rapidly. Now you can think or say what you want, but I can assure you, life can get very real, very quickly.

While I was lying in bed for so many days, unable to rise and getting worse instead of better, losing weight and feeling weak, my parents were full of anguish and concern. Papa would urge me to repent and get saved so I could go to heaven. I didn't fully know what it meant to repent or get saved, and I certainly didn't want to go to heaven at that time.

The fact was that Papa knew I was facing certain death, and he wanted his baby boy to be in a condition for his soul to go to heaven when his body died. He wanted the circle to be unbroken in heaven for his family.

Mama would say, "Oral, pray, pray." And I remember saying, "I don't know how to pray, Mama." This went on until one morning, she said in a bright tone of voice, "Oh, Son, you don't have to know how to pray. Just open your heart and talk to God as you would to me or to Papa. Tell Him you are sorry for rejecting Him, then believe He hears you. God will do the rest."

Although I didn't respond that day, I heard what she said. It hit home and made a lot of sense.

Now somehow, the Scriptures my parents poured into me came flooding over me. Hope and expectation began to fill my soul.

My miraculous healing was primed by seven words of faith from my sister Jewel. She marched into my room as I lay sick in bed, pointed her finger at me, and said, "Oral, God is going to heal you." I remember feeling hopeless and asking her, "Is He, Jewel?" Her words tumbled through my mind over the coming weeks and sparked my faith, paving the way for miracles in my life.

In 1935, a healing evangelist named George Moncey was holding services in Ada, Oklahoma. My brother Elmer was totally convinced that if he could bring me to the service to be prayed over, my body would be healed. He borrowed a car, placed a feather mattress in the back, and drove all the way from Ada to Stratford, Oklahoma, where we lived at the time. I remember looking out the window of my room, seeing the car and the mattress, but mostly seeing Elmer full of enthusiasm and expectation for what God was going to do in my life and in my body. Elmer came into the house with boldness. He didn't even say hello; he simply got me dressed, placed me on the mattress in the back of the car, and we all started back to Ada. He was in a hurry to get me to the meeting.

When we got there, I was carried into the meeting. About two hundred people lined up for prayer, and I was the last person to be prayed for. George Moncey came over and told me to stand up. I stood. The preacher placed his hands on my head and began to pray. I sat back down, and the preacher began to walk away. He paused. "Oral, come to me again." He prayed again and spoke the most positive prayer I had ever heard. There wasn't a doubt in his mind or his speech or his manner. He knew God wanted to impart healing to my emaciated body. *He knew it.* Touching my head with his hands, he did not plead with God. He did not ask if it was God's will for me to live. Instead, he took command over the sickness, saying, "You foul tormenting disease, I command you in the name of Jesus Christ of Nazareth to loose this boy. … Loose him, and let him go free!"

In that instant, I felt my faith being released and God's Spirit coming upon me. Suddenly, I whirled out of the hands of my parents who were on either side of me, holding me up, and cried, "I can breathe! I can breathe all the way down!" Gulping in great bursts of air, I was beside myself with joy. No more coughing, hemorrhaging, or pain. I felt free! Healing had taken place in my spirit and body! I ran onto the platform. Walking up and down the stage, I began to preach to the audience. As I began to tell what was happening, my words were free, and the stuttering stopped. I was healed in my speech as well as my body.

HEALED BUT STILL BATTLING

We returned home and that night, I was exhausted. For days and weeks afterward, I was very weak. I was healed, but the battle wasn't over. I began to doubt that God had healed me. Several days after the meeting, I remember lying outside on my cot—the outdoor tuberculosis patient *sickbed* of the time—and feeling discouraged. Having no strength, I felt as though death was looming over me. I asked my mother, "Do you believe that God healed me?" She responded confidently, "Yes, Son, I do." I had so many questions. "If the Lord healed me, why can't I get up and get around better? I thought if the Lord healed you, He healed you!" My mother was a woman of great faith. Looking intently at me, she said, "Yes, sometimes you are healed instantly. Other times you are healed, and your body begins to mend from a certain moment. Your recovery follows a normal course. In either case, you are healed by God's power, and it is wonderful." This profound statement changed my perspective on God's healing power. She continued, "You have had tuberculosis for a long time, and it took you many months to become weak. It will probably take you a while to regain your strength now that you are healed."

I didn't like that answer. I wanted to be up walking and running. Instead, I had to stand firm in my faith and continue standing day by day, sometimes reminding myself hour by hour that I had been healed by God. I absolutely received a healing touch, but I still had to gain weight and get my strength back. My greatest faith builder was my mother. She would consistently remind me, "Son, you stood up inside. Now keep standing. You began walking. Now keep walking."

WALKING IN HEALING

Slowly I began to regain my strength. I gained weight, my breathing eased, and my health seemed to improve each day. Finally, the day came when the doctor's report declared, "No tuberculosis found in this patient!" It was a miracle, and my house and the community were filled with rejoicing.

As I grew in strength, I began taking walks, eventually walking to town and back. One day, I was returning home from one of these walks when a woman ran out to me. "Are you Oral Roberts? The boy who was healed? My baby is dying. Please come and pray for him. God has healed you, and if you pray, I know God will heal my child!" I went into the woman's home, prayed for her dying baby, and the child was healed. The story spread all over town. This moment was not the beginning of my ministry. *It was the first fruit of it.* My healing ministry began with my parents on bended knee at my bedside, crying out for God to save me. I know that without their prayers and faith, I would never have become a healing evangelist who prayed for thousands. Because of their steadfast example of faith, I know that God will do what He says He will. I will forever be grateful for the faith builders and contenders of faith in my life.

"Rise, take up thy bed, and walk" (John 5:8). These were some of the most exciting words in the world when I was desperate for God's miraculous healing power, desperation that I knew well. I breath today through lungs that were once eaten up with tuberculosis. I speak through lips once bound by stuttering. I live a life that was once without meaning or relationship with God. I minister with an unshakable conviction of God's healing power and the knowledge from God that *"all things are possible to him who believes"* (Mark 9:23 NKJV).

2

PREACHING THE GOODNESS OF GOD

From that moment on, I walked with excitement in my heart. I had been healed, and I wanted to share that with everyone around me. However, I found out very quickly that not everyone shared that excitement. I learned that being healed did not necessarily mean being accepted. In my mind, I felt like once I was healed, I would return to a normal life. But the tuberculosis diagnosis meant that I would forever be an outcast to some, no matter how many "clear" reports the doctors issued.

I thought that if I could preach about the goodness of God and His healing power, the intense struggling that I had gone through up to that point would be over. And even though it was a completely different kind of struggle, nothing could be further from the truth. The Bible says Satan comes to steal, kill, and destroy (John 10:10), and I was his target, regardless of how the hits came.

As I studied the Bible, the Scripture came alive to me that says I would see the *"goodness of the LORD in the land of the living"*

(Psalm 27:13), but when I spoke about God's goodness and power to heal, some people thought I had turned against God or committed an unpardonable sin. They were not used to hearing that God was a healer or that God was good. I was raised on a gospel that believed in healing, and once I was healed, I had a firsthand, front-row seat to the goodness of God. For making statements like these, I was branded as a heretic and a fraud. People said I was a man who practiced medicine without a license and so much more. Most of these comments came from the church—the people who were supposed to be my greatest supporters, fellow brothers and sisters in Christ!

One time after I was healed, I was invited to preach at a small church in a neighboring town. The pastor who invited me believed my healing testimony. He was not afraid of me, even though I had previously been diagnosed with terminal tuberculosis. However, not everyone was so confident of my healing. It was planned for me to stay in the home of one of the church members, to save the expense of a hotel. As soon as I arrived at their home, the wife was excited to hear my testimony, but the husband was not. This man did not believe in healing; he thought that I was making the entire thing up and still carrying tuberculosis in my body. He must have thought I would infect his family.

It was a cold, snowy night, yet this man sent me out the door, into the snow, to walk to the nearest hotel. The cold was unbearable, but it could not compare to the coldness I felt in my heart for being rejected and ridiculed. I believed in the goodness of God and His healing power, and now I had to convince God's people that He wanted good things for them. He wanted to heal them, just as He did me. Nothing had prepared me for that rejection, especially from a church member.

I quickly came to understand that not every person, not every church member, would accept God as a good God, nor would they accept His healing power. But regardless of people's opinions, from that moment forward, my testimony became the foundation of my ministry. I allowed God to use my story to bring others a tangible revelation of His goodness and hope for healing.

MIRACLES AND MINISTRY

I spent time pastoring in several states and preparing for what God planned to do in my life. During those years, I met a young woman named Evelyn at a church camp meeting. We sat next to each other in the youth orchestra that night. I remember leaning over and asking her if my hair was combed. She replied, "Yes, it is. You look nice." Later that evening after the service, she wrote in her diary, "Tonight I met the man I will marry."

Evelyn was a schoolteacher who taught English in South Texas and had come back to Oklahoma for a vacation. She and I began corresponding by letters. For almost two years, we wrote back and forth to each other. She was such a good writer, and I think I began falling in love with her through those letters.

I decided to drive down to the Harlingen, Texas, area where she was teaching to see her. My mother wanted to go with me. She knew the call of God that was on my life and wanted to make certain in her own mind that Evelyn fit within that calling.

On that visit, I proposed to Evelyn in a most unusual way. I said to her, "My huge, happy, hilarious heart is throbbing tumultuously, tremendously, triumphantly, in a lasting long-lived love for you. As I gaze into your beauteous, bounteous, beaming eyes, I am literally lost in a daring, delightful dream in which your fair, felicitous, fancy-filled face is ever present like a colossal comprehensive constellation. Will you be my sweet, smiling, soulful, satisfied spouse?"

She replied, "Listen here, if you're trying to propose to me, talk in the English language." We laughed together and she accepted my proposal, which I sealed with a kiss. We were married that year on Christmas Day. From that moment on, she was my greatest source of uplifting prayer and support. I referred to her as *my darling wife Evelyn* every day until she went home to be with the Lord.

THE BEGINNING OF A WORLDWIDE MINISTRY

Just after my twenty-ninth birthday, the Holy Spirit brought about an abrupt change in my ministry. I had prayed for a man who had been injured. When he was healed, I was as astonished as he was. I had known that someday I would have a ministry of healing, but I kept asking, "When? Where? How?"

While pastoring in Toccoa, Georgia, one of our deacons named Clyde had an accident and I was called to pray for him. My associate, Bill, was in the room when I got the call, and he went with me. When we got there, Clyde was down on the ground, holding his right foot in his hands. He had dropped a heavy motor on it, which crushed his toes. He was in such pain that he was screaming at the top of his voice. All he could do was point to his foot, signifying that he wanted us to pray. As I looked down at him holding his foot, a sudden compassion came over me. Without thinking, I knelt down and touched the end of his shoe with my hand. I said a few words of earnest prayer and stood up.

The moment I stood up, Clyde quit screaming. He tried to move his toes in his shoe and found that he could do so. The pain was gone. Jumping to his feet, he stomped his foot on the floor and said, "Brother Roberts, what did you do to me?" I said, "Clyde, I didn't do a thing." He said, "Yes, you did. The pain is gone. My foot is healed." I was amazed. While I watched him, he stooped down, tore off his shoe, and showed us his foot. It was perfectly normal. I could not deny that a miracle had been wrought. When we left, Bill said, "Brother Roberts, do you have that kind of power all the time?" I said, "Bill, I wish I did." He said, "If you had that kind of power all the time, you could bring a revival to this world."

I thought a lot about what Bill said. He was right. When the power of the Lord comes upon a man to deliver the people, God brings revival to mankind.

Not long after that, Evelyn and I left Toccoa and returned to Oklahoma. It was in Enid that God spoke to me a second time. Some of the best people in the world were members of the church; they loved me, and I had a wonderful ministry among them. About fifty new people joined the church during this time and it looked as if I was going to have the best ministry of my life there.

It was about this time that I began to be reminded of the voice of God that I had heard twelve years before. I would start to get up and preach at the church when I would hear the Lord say, "You are to take My healing power to your generation."

I would be sitting in the classroom and I would hear God say, "You are to take My healing power to your generation." I would be out with a group of the church men hunting or fishing, and God would say, "You are to take My healing power to your generation." I would be studying my Bible to preach when I would hear God say, "You are to take My healing power to your generation." I could not get away from His voice to me.

GOD'S ANOINTING TO PRAY FOR THE SICK

One thought became dominant in my mind: "I must have God's anointing to pray for the sick." I knew there would be many difficulties, serious criticisms, and unhappy misunderstandings. I knew also that I, as a human being, would be subject to failures and mistakes. And I realized that the ministry of healing through prayer for the sick was a departure from the other ministries commonly known at that time and would require unusual qualities in the man God chose to use.

With all these things striving together within me, I reached the point of no return. I found my only desire was to make contact with the Lord so I might hear His voice again and receive my instructions.

People around me knew something was about to happen, and some of them would not let me alone. I found I was being hindered in my search for God. One morning, I told Evelyn I was going to remain in prayer until the Lord revealed Himself to me. She smiled encouragingly and promised to be much in prayer herself.

I told the Lord I had come to the end of myself and that I would not leave Him until He spoke to me.

It is said that when a man makes up his mind, he never changes. My mind was made up. The hours of meditation, study, and prayer had brought me to this point. The die was cast, and my future was set. Now I was prepared to receive the mighty touch of God's hand.

I felt the need to fast and pray. I have no idea how long I prayed. In my intensity and concentration, I virtually lost sight of time and space. I hardly knew who I was or where I was. In a sense, I felt like a speck in the universe as I poured out my soul to the Lord. Slowly, almost imperceptibly, I felt myself drawn closer and closer to God. I became conscious that I was praying in the Spirit and that the Spirit had control of me. Somewhere in the prayer, I had the feeling that my struggling and striving were over, that Jesus was standing by my side. I felt something going out of me and something coming into me.

Suddenly, God spoke to me in an audible voice. He spoke like a military commander, words of crisp command, clear and strong: "Stand upon your feet." I stood and found myself facing the door. "Go and get in your car." In the car, I sat with my hands upon the wheel.

Then God said, "Drive one block and turn right." As I turned the corner, God said, "From this hour, your ministry of healing will begin. You will have My healing power to pray for the sick and to cast out devils."

Beginning at the pit of my stomach, an exhilaration was rising in me, and I was flooded with indescribable joy. I began to praise God aloud, and I noticed a new vibrancy and authority in my voice, which I never had before, and which has been with me ever since.

I drove home, dashed into the house, found Evelyn, and hugged her to me. I said, "You can cook now!"—meaning my fast was over.

She said, "Oral, the Lord has spoken to you, hasn't He?"

I asked her, "How did you know?"

She smiled, "By looking at you, of course!"

Heretofore I had prayed for the sick as a normal and usual part of my ministry. A few had been healed, but not all of them. From this hour, however, I was entering into God's special call in the ministry of healing. As some ministers are especially called to teach, I was especially called to pray for the sick. Hence, I would particularly emphasize this phase of the gospel in my preaching, and in this emphasis, my ministry was to be different from the preaching and ministry of other people. They would do their par-ticular work, and I would do mine.

I decided to make a test to prove to myself that God had truly spoken to me. I realize now that my action was rather daring—and perhaps foolish—but it must be remembered that I felt I had to know beyond any shadow of doubt. I planned to conduct a public service in Enid and to invite the sick to come for prayer. I had been preaching in my church to a congregation of approximately two hundred people. I asked the Lord for three things in that first ser-vice: first, to give me an audience of a thousand people; second, to supply the financial needs; and third, to heal the people by divine power so conclusively that they, as well as I, would know I was called of God in this special ministry.

I promised God, "Lord, if you will grant these three things, I will resign my pastorate and enter immediately into evangelistic crusades."

I secured the use of the lovely auditorium in the Educational Building in downtown Enid for 2:00 p.m. the following Sunday and gave out announcements for the meeting. God performed my three requests. An accurate count of the crowd revealed that more than 1,200 persons were present; the freewill offering met the rental, advertising, and other costs with about three dollars left over; and after the sermon, God did show His miracle-working power in healing and delivering the people.

The title of my sermon was, "If You Need Healing, Do These Things!" The anointing of the Holy Spirit was so strong upon me that my flesh quivered. The vibrancy and authority I had noticed in my voice after God spoke to me were present again, and almost immediately, my audience and I were one. I felt at home, preaching to the largest congregation I had ever addressed in Enid. My old fear was gone, and through the anointing of God, my soul was afire. I found a love in my heart for those people. I wanted to touch them, to pray for them, to help them in their needs.

The people felt this, and before I had finished preaching—as if by a prearranged signal—they rose to their feet and stood before me. I sensed it was God's time to heal and that the people were ready and expectant. I walked down from the platform to the aisle on my left, next to the wall. About three hundred people thronged into the aisle and came in a long line to meet me.

The first person in the line was a woman from a nearby German settlement. She told me she had had a stiff hand for thirty-eight years. I laid my right hand upon her head and prayed for her healing in the name of Jesus of Nazareth. Instantly, she cried out at the top of her voice that she was healed, lifting up her stiff hand and opening and closing it for all to see. God had taken away the stiffness and given her perfect use of the hand. Several others were healed by God in quick succession, and it greatly helped the faith of the audience.

Three men walked over to me and said, "We are not sick, but we need to be saved. After seeing all this, we want to give our hearts to God." I prayed with them, and the Lord saved their souls. For the next two hours, I prayed alternately with the sick and the unsaved. When it was over and I stood alone, drenched in perspiration, I watched the people leave. I had prayed until there was scarcely a dry thread in my clothes. I was supposed to be exhausted; instead, I felt strong.

My proof was before me! Not everyone I prayed for had been healed, even as not all are healed today. But the people who were there knew God was with me, and best of all, I knew it too—and would know it forever!

We had agreed to hold a tent revival in Tulsa for Pastor Steve Pringle. The service in his tent opened in a driving rainstorm, with a small crowd. Compared with the huge tents we used later in my ministry, that tent was very small, but at the time it was the biggest one I had seen in use for the gospel. It seated over 1,400 people. From the moment I had opened my mouth, I was conscious of the anointing of the Holy Spirit, and I was able to preach with the fire and power of God upon me. There were a few sick people present, and we had a prayer line for them. Some of them felt that they had been definitely and miraculously healed. Several others were converted to Christ on that opening night. It seemed that within hours, the news had spread like fire over Tulsa. Within three nights, the tent was packed. On Sunday, the place was not only filled, but there were hundreds standing around the edges of the tent. Pastor Pringle said, "Okay, Oral, you can't close this meeting. God is with you, and you must stay another week." The revival continued for nine straight weeks and was standing room only.

One evening, I was praying for a blind man who had been brought from Kansas. Suddenly he screamed, "I can see! I can see!" Excitement ran like electricity through the audience. People stood up and cried like children, giving thanks to God. I remember telling God that I had dreamed of an hour like this and that if He would continue blessing me, I would spend the rest of my life praying for the healing of the sick and winning souls to Christ.

As the meeting continued, the tent was usually filled two or three hours before the nightly services began. Many of the fine pastors of Tulsa dismissed their weeknight services and helped us. There was a unity among the people who attended, although they were from different churches and walks of life. I was now beginning to see what this ministry could do to bring people together. It blotted out all denominational barriers and disunity. As I stood up each evening to preach, I felt the greatest anointing I had ever known. I preached for an hour and a half in each service, and the people were seemingly spellbound. God opened the Scriptures of deliverance to me when I preached of His goodness and His power.

A DIFFERENT BRUSH WITH DEATH

It was in this Tulsa crusade that I had my first brush with death as an evangelist of God. One night when I was preaching, a man whom none of us knew stood on the opposite side of the street. He stood there a few minutes, pulled out a revolver, pointed it in my general direction, and pulled the trigger. The bullet plowed through the canvas tent about eighteen inches above my head. The people heard the gunshot, but providentially, no one paid any attention to it.

The next day, I saw the bullet hole. Standing there, I wondered if what was meant for my harm benefitted me instead. I asked God to give me courage and divine protection until I had finished my work. The news wire services headlined the shooting incident throughout the nation and around the world. Overnight, I was labeled a famous controversial evangelist. I did not know the meaning of this experience at that early stage of my ministry, but I now know that it helped pave the way for me to keep my balance and perspective.

The gunman probably had no idea why he shot at me that night. His action was unlike the planned and organized persecution that I was to face again and again. In those times, when I was in the midst of such severe persecution, I would remember the incident in Steve Pringle's tent and recalled that it happened during my first crusade of deliverance. Because it was an unusual event, I'm sure that God was trying to show me that my life would be composed of positives and negatives, and that we are often locked in unusual spiritual combat (Ephesians 6:12).

3

OPENING UP TO GOD

I believe the greatest miracle in life is the saving of a person's soul. There are several terms for this, including "getting saved," "receiving forgiveness of sins," "being born again," and "having personal salvation."

I've gone through this myself. I've gone through it with thousands of others and still do.

Speaking very frankly, I believe getting your soul saved and continuing a salvation lifestyle can lead you to what I have so often said is the greatest miracle you will ever experience.

The saving of your soul is the saving of *you*. It is your own personal salvation given to you from God. You are very important, and Jesus says, *"Ye must be born again"* (John 3:7).

No *if* or *hope so* or *maybe so*—you must!

Salvation is available to everyone, and God wants everyone to have it. Second Peter 3:9 says, *"The Lord is not slack concerning his promise, as some men count slackness; but is long-suffering to us-ward, not willing that any should perish, but that all should come to repentance."*

Miracles of healing and other miracles are not accidents, although some people may appear to have health when their lifestyle is against God. But He wants us to have better health and miracle-living, which involve much more than physical health. I'm talking about total well-being—in the now ... and forever.

FIRST THINGS FIRST

Jesus said, *"It is better for you to enter life lame, rather than having two feet, to be cast into hell, into the fire that shall never be quenched"* (Mark 9:45 NKJV).

This passage describes the severity of sin and the importance of dealing with it readily. Jesus doesn't mean that your body or your soul are not important, but He seeks to help you put your priorities in the right order. First things first.

Jesus is encouraging His listeners to prioritize their spiritual well-being above all else, emphasizing the importance of avoiding sin at all costs. In Scripture, He tells you that your spirit is the most important part of you, and the healing and restoration of the spirit from the disease of sin is the most important healing.

WHEN I TURNED AWAY FROM GOD

A false picture of a life saved from sin presented itself to my mind. My strong dream of becoming a lawyer and, ultimately, governor of Oklahoma seemed totally unattainable if I were to become a saved person, so I turned off all feelings for God. However, He didn't turn off His feelings for me. I still felt that tugging feeling inside that I should admit I was a sinner, I should ask for God's forgiveness and for personal salvation. But I didn't ask because I didn't want to. I didn't feel the need to.

I remember one day, it was like God and I were in a room all alone. In my imagination, I was facing Him. I felt crowded, uncomfortable, resentful, and cheated that what I was dreaming might never happen. Crushed in my spirit over it, I shouted, "God, get out of my life! Let me alone!"

GOD LET ME ALONE

I thought that ended it since I felt a sort of release. As time wore on, I slowly became aware of something happening inside me. *God had gotten out of my life. He **had** left me alone.*

At first, I thought, "Great!" Then it wasn't so good. It was an eerie kind of feeling.

God had let me be on my own, to go it alone. Now, strangely, I wasn't so sure I wanted it like this. I began to have an awareness about life and death; I considered what would happen if a sinner died versus what would happen if a Christian died.

As a young man, it hadn't occurred to me that young people died. That was something that happened to the very old. My grandfather Roberts had died at age eighty-four, but that was an age many times my own, and it seemed like an eternity away from my present years.

DO YOU NEED A NEW LIFE?

Two things happened that brought me to a decision to repent and turn to Christ. These two things may seem unique to me, but I believe they really aren't, as you will see.

At that time, I had made no connection between being saved from sin and being healed of tuberculosis or stammering. In the thinking of most people I knew, there was quite a separation spiritually between the saving of the soul and a cure or healing coming to one's physical body. You prayed to God for your soul, and you went to the doctor for your body. Better health and miracle living didn't seem to go with salvation. The possibility of miracles was viewed as foolish and impractical. Little to none of it was taught either in the church or in medical circles that I was aware of.

In a way, it didn't seem to be a good time to get saved, nor a good time to turn myself over to doctors. The distance and misunderstanding between them seemed great, and I was caught in the middle. Both were extremely important, but I felt like they needed only to get a little closer together, especially for people like me who urgently needed both.

I WASN'T GOING TO MAKE IT

The first thing I realized when I was diagnosed with tuberculosis was that I wasn't going to make it. So if what my parents told me about my need of God and God's willingness to save me were true, then I should get serious about it.

The sense of sin (or the sense of rejecting God) had not fully hit me, and I discovered that without it, I couldn't concede I was a sinner. This was taken care of in an unexpected way. While my parents gathered near my bed in family prayer, with the burden of their prayer for me, I looked up into Papa's face and what appeared to me in his countenance turned me around.

I thought I saw Jesus Christ in my father's face. The image of Christ shone and my mind, through my eyes, saw it. I burst into tears. That apparent vision of the Man of Galilee was so real to my senses that involuntarily I called out, "O God, come into my life; save my soul." The sense of sin was on me unexplainably but clear. Moments later, the presence of God came over me. I felt that God accepted me as I accepted Him; I felt new and renewed inside.

OPENING YOUR MIND TO CHRIST

Having a need and seeing something of Christ in another person that gives one a personal sense of his sins or separation from God are the two things I believe must happen *before anyone is willing* to think seriously about getting saved or receiving what we know as salvation.

When I say, "having a need," I don't necessarily mean a need like mine, a direct need for physical healing. Nor do I mean one has to have some kind of spiritual vision of Christ as I did. But I believe everybody has a need and everybody will have some experience of God in the Person of Christ that is real to them. The *way* it happens is not as important as that it *does* happen. In other words, when you open your mind to Christ, He can make Himself known to you. You can depend on it happening—to you.

THE OLD SHEPHERD SAW THE GLORY

Getting to know Christ is like the summer day when a great scientist went up into the Scottish mountains to study a particular flower that was blooming at that time in all its glory. He wanted to look at it through his microscope without picking it to see it in all its perfection. He knelt down, adjusted his microscope, and soon was reveling in the flower's delicate color and beauty.

He was still in this position a few minutes later when a shadow fell across him. Looking up, he saw an old Highland shepherd watching him. Without saying a word, the scientist picked the flower and handed it, with the microscope, to the shepherd so that he too could see the beautiful sight. As the old shepherd looked, tears began streaming down his face. Then, handing the flower back very tenderly, he said, "Man, I wish you'd never shown me that."

"Why?" asked the scientist, puzzled.

"Because," he said, "these rude feet of mine have trodden on them so many times."

Just as the old shepherd encountered the flower's beauty, I believe something like this can happen to you concerning Christ and His glory for your life. I pray that's when you, like me, will want to get a new spiritual heart.

A HEART TRANSPLANT

The first time I was on the Johnny Carson television show, I followed a special guest, the famous heart transplant surgeon, Dr. Christiaan Barnard of South Africa. In the interview, Mr. Carson asked Dr. Barnard to share his most exciting experience in relation to his work.

Dr. Barnard said, "I believe the greatest experience of all happened one day as I was making a postoperative checkup on one of my patients. He said, 'Doctor, I wonder if you would let me see my old heart. I think it would help my attitude.' It was an unusual request, but I consented. Soon attendants wheeled in a big cart on which was a glass jar containing the man's heart."

Dr. Barnard said, "I took my pen and pointed to the problem area of his old heart. I told him, 'This is what would have killed you if you hadn't received a new heart.' The patient looked up and said with such gratitude, 'Doc, I'm so grateful you took out that old heart that was killing me and gave me a new heart!'"

That line expresses so aptly the joy I felt at age seventeen when I received a new heart—a spiritual transformation—from the Great Physician, Jesus Christ!

My new spiritual heart meant my spirit was reborn. The term, "responding first through your spirit," had not come to me then, but I've come to learn that's exactly what I did. From deep within, I felt hope that I would live and not die with the disease that was destroying me. The gospel of Jesus Christ faithfully imparted by my parents to me over the years finally paid off—in a big way.

I believe the hardest part of this is to become aware that you need to be saved, to admit you are a sinner, and that you are saved only by the Person of Jesus Christ. This begins with feeling a sense of sin.

HOW TO DEAL WITH SIN IN YOUR LIFE

You will hear me say again and again, God's greatest miracle is the salvation of a soul.

We hear people say:

+ "The operation saved me."
+ "I was in an accident, but I was saved."
+ "I came out of it and now everything is going to be all right."

When people say such things, I think they mean they have been saved by coming through some bad incident. But what I'm talking about is much more than that. I mean the saving of your soul, your inner self made in the image and likeness of God. Your spirit, through your faith, is your direct, inner connection to God in order to experience the salvation of your soul. Really, it's your total self being saved.

So as you become aware of a sense of sin in your life, I want you to consider speaking these four statements aloud and thinking about how they can apply to you:

1. I am aware of my need for a new life in Christ.

2. I will pray that I will see Christ reflected in another person's life.

3. I want to be aware of a sense of sin and do something about it to bring full healing to my whole person.

4. In my healing process, I will begin practicing forgiveness because this opens me up to healing.

I believe it's vital that you receive a renewed spiritual life. In addition to being born as a natural being, *"You must be born again,"* as Jesus told Nicodemus in John 3:7 (NKJV). He is still saying this to you and me! Before you go further into this book, I want to give you the opportunity to know Him as Savior and Lord and be born again so you will have solid ground on which to claim the promises of His Word. Let's look at the steps involved in being born again and entering into a new life in Christ.

STEPS TO BEING BORN AGAIN

In leading someone to Jesus, I've always said there are four steps to being born again: reaching the point that you recognize your need for a Savior; telling God you want Him as your Savior and your source of supplying your needs; receiving Christ as Lord; and recognizing the work of the Holy Spirit in the new birth. Let's look at each step individually.

1. Reach the point that you recognize you need a Savior.

The need for a Savior comes from the Scripture that says, *"All have sinned, and come short of the glory of God"* (Romans 3:23).

We need to recognize that like everyone else on earth, people do sin at times; if you don't recognize sin, it can lead you into becoming a sinner who makes sin a lifestyle. Without a change, you can carry your sins into death and into the eternal judgment. If you do this, you can miss the opportunity to enjoy eternity with God. This will not be God's choice, since He gave His only begotten Son, Jesus, that you should be saved and not be lost. It will be your own choice if you reject Him.

My realization that I was a sinner was my first step to God. It led me to the sinner's prayer: *"God be merciful to me a sinner"* (Luke 18:13). In that moment, I prayed those words and asked Christ to save me.

Let's look at the background of these simple, life-changing words, *"God be merciful to me a sinner,"* found in the parable Jesus told in Luke 18:9–14:

> *And he spake this parable unto certain which trusted in themselves that they were righteous, and despised others: two men went up into the temple to pray; the one a Pharisee, and the other a publican. The Pharisee stood and prayed thus with himself, God, I thank thee, that I am not as other men are, extortioners, unjust, adulterers, or even as this publican. I fast twice in the week, I give tithes of all that I possess. And the publican, standing afar off, would not lift up so much as his eyes unto heaven, but smote upon his breast, saying, God be merciful to me a sinner. I tell you, this man went down to his house justified rather than the other: for every one that exalteth himself shall be abased; and he that humbleth himself shall be exalted.*

The publican, a tax collector, recognized his need for a Savior. He knew his only hope was in God's mercy. When a person reaches this point, whether it happened centuries ago, as in this parable, or whether it happens for you today, God hears, answers, and saves.

2. Tell God you want Him as your Savior, as your Source.

When you desire to know God as your Savior and Source, you can tell Him this sincerely when you recognize that you need Him, that only *He* can save you and be the Source of your total supply. Telling God you want Him as your Savior and Source is important. The apostle Paul writes in Romans 10:9, *"If thou shalt **confess**

with thy mouth the Lord Jesus, and shalt believe in thine heart that God hath raised him from the dead, thou shalt be saved."

I believe wanting God is a process of understanding your need for Him. Once you understand you need Him, you can come to understand the importance of making Him your Source. It's allowing Him to become the guiding light of your spirit.

3. Receive Christ in your heart.

Receive Jesus Christ as a Person. *Receiving* in this sense is different from getting. It's a little more difficult, in a way, to receive. Saying "I'll get this guy," or "I'll get this thing," or "I'll get this deal" is not the same as, "I'll receive Christ into my heart as my personal Savior and Source."

When you receive, you also give. What do you give? You give your sins to God, and you give Him all your past mistakes. You give Him today. Then you can determine to give Him your entire future. Your start is a one-time thing, but your continuing is more, a continuous series of loving by giving Him the essence of your life. In doing so, you can look to find new ways to love or give of yourself. This is true seed-faith living.

It's in this spirit of giving to Him that your seed of faith is planted, and from this planting, you can *receive*. You receive the living Christ, the greatest miracle of all. He comes into your heart, to your soul, and you receive Him not as a guest but as your Savior, Lord, and your Source.

For me, the most helpful aspect of having given myself and my sins to God is that I meant it. The start I made at seventeen was a real decision I made. It was something I felt to the core of my being. It was no flash-in-the-pan kind of thing. The sinner had been changed to a Christian.

The Bible says when you and I receive Christ as our Lord and Savior, we are spiritually remade and reborn in His image and likeness, thus the term *"born again"* in John 3:3. Being a Christian means we can carry Him in our hearts throughout life and into death, given the opportunity to live in heaven and life with Him forever.

4. Recognize the work of the Holy Spirit in the process of Christ giving you a new birth.

In the process of being born again, the remade new birth, Christ receives you to Himself and brings Himself to you, saving your soul. This makes you a new creation in Christ—removing old things such as sins and the old nature that is unlike God—so that all things become new and pure in Him (2 Corinthians 5:17).

Who is the Holy Spirit? He is the *"Comforter"* (John 14:16), the One whom Christ said He would send to us to replace His own physical presence on earth. The Holy Spirit is God coming to us in His own spiritual, invisible, unlimited form to live *in* you and to abide *with* you forever (John 14:16–17).

You see, God is one God. Deuteronomy 6:4 tells us, *"The Lord our God is one Lord."* When we call Him Father, Son, and Holy Spirit—the Holy Trinity—we are not saying He is three Gods. He is simply God: God manifesting Himself as the *Father* with a specific work to do, as the *Son* with a specific work to do, and as the *Holy Spirit* with a specific work to do.

Let's use water as a simple example of how to think about the Holy Trinity. It's always water but it can manifest or express itself three ways: at room temperature as liquid; frozen as ice; and as steam or vapor when boiled. But it is still water, used in different ways as the need arises.

As an expression of God's love for us, the *Father* sent the *Son, Jesus Christ*, to earth be born of a woman. He sent Him to become a human being for at least three reasons:

1. The Father—*El-Elyon*, the Most High—is the creator and possessor of heaven and earth. He is loving, good, and kind, our Abba or Daddy. His love for us is so great and personal that He wants us to be healed and whole (Genesis 14:19; John 5:20; 14:9; 1 John 4:16).

2. The Father sent the Son, Jesus, to sit where we sit, feel what we feel, go through all we experience, and show us the way through it (John 3:16–17; Hebrews 4:15). In the greatest act of giving the world has ever known, the Father sent the Son to give Himself as the divine seed on the cross for our sins. That seed became the miracle harvest of the resurrection so that we, too, can live forever in heaven with Jesus (John 3:16; 11:25–26; Galatians 3:16; Ephesians 2:13–18).

3. After Jesus Christ, the Son, was crucified and raised from the dead, He ascended to heaven and prayed to the Father to send the Holy Spirit. Thus, the Spirit of God manifested as the Holy Spirit, not in the form of the Son in flesh but as the Spirit He inherently is, who comes into our spirit to lead, guide, and comfort us (John 4:24).

Remember, God originally made man a spirit. He didn't make him just a soul or a body only. He made him a living soul placed within a body.

Through the indwelling Holy Spirit, the unlimited form of God comes to dwell within your spirit. He's your inner man, your connection with God. With Him, you are in a position to enter into miracle-living for your total being.

As a Christian, I've always believed that seeking health is limiting. I don't seek health; instead, I seek God who is the Source of all, not only of my health but of my entire being, my entire life. For me, I don't see a doctor expecting him to be the source of my health. God is my Source; the doctor is one of the instruments God uses for health, and medicine is one of God's delivery systems for my health care. But I believe the Source of both—the skill of the doctor and the healing properties of medicine—*is God*!

As a Christian in need of healing, I had to get this point clear in my mind—that I started with God as my Source and then sought the help of His instruments such as prayer, medicine, doctors, etc. or a combination of them all. Then I could be on the right road to better health in every aspect of my life—spiritually, physically, financially, in my relationships, or in my work.

WHAT DOES IT MEAN TO BE BORN AGAIN?

When you are born again, you belong to the Father through receiving the work of the Son on the cross, by the power of the Holy Spirit. To be born again is to experience a spiritual rebirth, a transformation of the heart and soul that brings you into a new relationship with God. It is not merely a religious ritual or intellectual assent to certain beliefs, but a profound encounter with God that changes the course of your life. The Bible says when you are born again, you become a child of God, belonging to the Father through the redemptive work of the Son on the cross, empowered by the Holy Spirit (John 3:3–17; Ephesians 2:4–9).

Being born again signifies a spiritual awakening, a recognition of our need for salvation and a surrender to the saving grace of Jesus Christ. It is a turning point, a moment of surrender and acceptance, whereby we acknowledge our sins and receive forgiveness and new life in Christ. Through faith in Jesus, we are reconciled to God, adopted into His family, and granted the assurance of eternal life.

The process of being born again is initiated by the Holy Spirit, who convicts us of sin, righteousness, and judgment, leading us to repentance and faith in Jesus Christ. It is through the power of the

Holy Spirit that we are transformed from the inside out, making us new creations in Christ.

A PRAYER OF SALVATION

If you are ready to accept Jesus as your Lord and Savior, please say this prayer of salvation:

> *Heavenly Father, I come before You, recognizing my need for Your saving grace. I confess my shortcomings and ask for Your forgiveness. I believe in Jesus Christ, Your Son, who died on the cross for my sins and rose again, offering me redemption and new life.*
>
> *Lord Jesus, I invite You into my heart and surrender my life to You. Fill me with Your Holy Spirit and guide me in Your ways. Wash away my sins and make me whole in Your sight.*
>
> *Thank You, Lord, for Your unfailing love and mercy. I commit to following You faithfully and sharing Your message of hope with others.*
>
> *In the mighty name of Jesus, I pray. Amen.*

4

IT'S NEVER TOO LATE TO
WALK WITH GOD

I believe salvation is for everyone at any point in life. It's never too late to begin a personal relationship with God through Jesus Christ. When that happens, whether a person is young or advanced in years, everything can change.

I read a book about a man who was nearly eighty-four years old and had faced adversity of almost every kind. He began his career as a laborer at a sawmill and became a giant in the furniture-making industry. He had many manufacturing plants and his thousands of employees had great affection for this man who provided them with work and a generous profit-sharing plan. His sons were outstanding men too—one was in public life, one headed the operations of the plants, and the others were also doing well.

This man was known for his generous spirit and was respected by many.

We had been getting letters from him for two or three years in which he stated appreciation for our television ministry. He said his inner life was inspired by my sermons and prayers both on television and in my books.

One day, I appeared in a certain area and as I walked into the building, a man said, "You're Oral Roberts, aren't you?"

I said, "Yes, I am."

"Well, there's a man on the phone here asking for you," he said as he handed me the receiver.

The voice on the other end said, "Oral Roberts?"

"Yes?"

"I am ..." and he told me his name.

"Yes?"

"You remember I've been writing to you for your prayers."

"I remember a person by that name, but I don't believe I have met you personally."

"You have not, and that is the object of my phone call. I feel elated I reached you like this since I had a hunch to call you at this phone, not knowing for sure if you would be there. But you are."

"What can I do for you?"

"You can pray for *me*."

"I've been doing that."

"Well, I'm only a short distance away and my son is standing by to drive me. Would you pray for me if I come over to you?"

"Certainly," I said, "just be here in about a half hour and we'll find a quiet corner for the prayer."

When we met, I saw a man who looked like a man of strength and courage. For his years, he appeared to be healthy. He said, "My back needs healing. The surgeons over the years have kept me going but they feel, and I feel, I'm going to need a special touch, a miracle as you call it. Would you help me?"

PRAYING IN FAITH

I pointed out that since I could not heal but was an instrument of our Lord's healing power, I wanted him to think particularly of Jesus's hands when we joined hands, and suggested we pray for one another.

"You mean you want me to pray for you?" he asked.

"Yes," I replied, "that's *planting a seed of your faith*. That's giving of your concern and faith for someone else, as the Bible teaches in James 5:16, 'Pray one for another that ye may be healed.' That is, the seed you plant in someone else's life is designed to come back to you in the form of your need. Then I will pray for you as a seed I plant and believe God will bless us both."

He said, "I would like very much to do as you ask: pray for you, and I do pray, but really, I don't feel I can pray effectively. You see, I want to be sure I am born again."

I immediately sensed this was the key issue. This was why he had come. His back was troubling him, and he knew I would be concerned for his healing. He knew deep within him that it was absolutely essential that he be born again by the Spirit of God and that he knew it beyond any doubt.

At age eighty-four, not even the vast achievements he had accomplished would suffice. He had heard me speak enough to know that I clearly believed that being born again is essential for better health and miracle-living at any age. I knew he could have both the new birth of salvation *and* help for his back, and I told him so. "God is interested in whole-person healing. Everything about you is important to Him."

As I reached my hands to his for the dual prayer—or what I call the seed-faith prayer—I saw the strained look on his face.

"Is there something else wrong?" I asked.

"Well, I ... I ... just want to be sure that I am born again. I've been troubled about it for a great many years. Your coming to this area brought it to the surface and I want it very much. ... I want the life our Lord promised ... I want life ..." His voice trailed off.

Abruptly, I said, "Please repeat after me the sinner's prayer which Jesus gave in Luke 18:13: *'Lord, be merciful to me a sinner.'"*

Slowly, with obvious deep feeling, he said, "Lord, be merciful to me ... to me ... a sinner."

GOD HEARS PRAYER

"Now," I said, "tell God you believe He heard you and you believe He receives you as a spiritually newborn child in His kingdom."

After he did so, he said, "This is so important to me. I've been so long wanting God to let me know I am born again. Now it's here."

We rejoiced together. "What about your back?"

"Oh, yes," he replied. "You think He will help me there too?"

"All of you is His. Your body is a temple of His Spirit, and you are to glorify God with your body as you do with your spirit and mind—with your whole self."

Then, I read to him from 1 Corinthians 6:19–20 (NKJV):

Do you not know that your body is the temple of the Holy Spirit who is in you, whom you have from God, and you are not your own? For you were bought at a price; therefore glorify God in your body and in your spirit, which are God's.

PRAYING AS A SEED

I said, "God wants you—the total you—to be in miracle living. I believe there's a miracle for your back just the same as for your soul being born again. Now let's join hands again and as you pray for me, make it a seed for God to multiply back in healing for your back."

After we prayed, he said, "This is some experience for me. I believe God has seen fit to answer my prayers. I've tried to be a good man, working hard and helping people. But this is a great difference."

I said, "Yes, it means your last years can be your best years by learning to live a seed-faith lifestyle."

He smiled and said, "Reverend Roberts, I've been reading and studying your seed-faith book for months now, and it is of immeasurable help to me. I never miss one of your telecasts."

On leaving, he said, "Being born again is important, isn't it?"

I said, "So important that Jesus said in John 3:3–5 that it is the only way you can see and enter the kingdom of God. I was born again at age seventeen and I feel it's just as important to me now as it was then—it means my life is in God, and I believe it means the same for you and everyone who wants abundant and eternal life."

I can still picture him as he got into the car, looking at me and waving as he was driven away. I can still see his beaming face. It said, "I am born again."

IN THE BIG CRUSADES

From 1947 through 1968, I conducted evangelistic crusades before large audiences throughout America and all the continents.

In every service, in every sermon, in every healing line, I would always say, "God's greatest miracle is the saving of your soul." It was true for the eighty-four-year-old man, and I believe is true for every human being.

Since 1968, when I felt God wanted me to concentrate most of my ministry on weekly television, plus quarterly prime-time specials, I have continued to say, "God's greatest miracle is the saving of your soul." Sometimes I use other phrases meaning the same thing: being born again, or God forgiving your sins, or accepting Christ as your personal Savior. These are synonymous terms meaning you are made a new creation in Jesus Christ. Second Corinthians 5:17 (NKJV) says: "*Therefore, if anyone is in Christ, he is a new creation; old things have passed away; behold, all things have become new.*"

YOU CAN CONNECT WITH GOD

You reach God through your soul, your mind, your will, and your emotions. To me, it's a choice you can make, a decision to yield these aspects of your being to Him.

When God breathed the breath of life into Adam's body, he became something more powerful, more valuable, and more responsible than any other living creature. He became "*a living soul*" (Genesis 2:7). Human beings are God's masterpieces.

This inbreathing of God's own spiritual and moral likeness into the physical body of mankind caused us to become spiritual beings. Because this is the way God made people, I believe it is so important for you and for me to respond to life *first through our spirit.* As spiritual beings, we must respond from what we are.

At the well in Samaria, Jesus declared to the woman who was a sinner, "*God is a Spirit: and they that worship him must worship him in spirit*" (John 4:24). *In spirit.*

God, who is Spirit, made you like Himself; therefore, your soul, your spirit, or your inner man must govern your physical and intellectual life. This is the whole-person approach that can lift you to the highest level of health and success in this life.

POINT OF CONTACT

You may recall that I heard voice of God tell me, "You are to take My healing power to your generation," not just once but several times. After that, He did use me to bring healing to people, but I did not understand how.

Then one night while I was in the prayer line in Oklahoma, God spoke to me again. What He said this time helped to fill a missing link between my ministry and the people seeking healing. A mother brought her small boy forward and told me that he was totally deaf in one ear and partially deaf in the other. She said he couldn't hear a voice either beside or behind him, but if you spoke distinctly and directly to him so that he could see you, he could hear reasonably well.

I started to put my hands upon the child's head and pray for him when I heard the voice of God as clearly as if He was standing beside me. God said, "Son, you have been faithful up to this time, and now you will feel My presence in your right hand." He told me I was to feel His presence in this manner as *a point of contact* and the people and I would be able to release our faith for His healing power. I have no idea how long I stood there with my hand stretched out toward the child. It must've been several moments because I remember the thought that went through my mind, "The point of contact. ... This is the thing I have been needing."

When I became conscious of my surroundings again, I was looking at my right hand and saying to myself, "If I really hear God's voice, and if this warmth which I feel in my hands is His presence, then I believe God will open this boy's ears." I placed my two hands upon the child's ears and immediately was aware of a warm feeling of God's presence in my right hand, but scarcely anything unusual in the left. There was a distinct difference. I prayed for a moment with my hands in this position, and then I touched the other side of the boy's head with my right hand.

I was so positive the Lord had touched the boy's ears and that he would be able to hear normally that I asked his mother to stand behind him and speak to him. She called him by name, and he whirled around to face her. Then I had the mother stand at his side, and he heard her clearly. When it dawned upon the mother and the child that he was healed, they started hugging each other while tears streamed down their cheeks. It was like being in the presence of God.

A little later, I went over to a woman who had not been able to walk without help for eight years because her body had grown very stiff with arthritis. She was seated where she could see and hear what had been going on. When I touched her in the name of Christ, I again felt this warmth in my right hand. I whispered to her, "Release your faith toward God now." The presence of the Lord came upon her; with a sudden movement, she rose from her chair and began walking and then running through the audience. It seemed as if the entire audience stood up with uplifted hands and praised God. Evelyn was nearby, and when I looked at her, her face shined like an angel's, as if she was ready to fly away in her happiness.

DIFFERENT POINTS OF CONTACT FROM GOD

The following day, I told Evelyn what God had said to me and how I felt the warmth of His presence for a few moments during the service. She said, "Oral, this is assigned to you." She reminded me that different men in the Bible were given a certain sign by God for their spiritual ability to help people. We talked over some of the signs such as Moses's rod, which became a point of contact for the releasing his faith as well as the people's; Samuel's horn of oil; David's slingshot; Peter's shadow; and the handkerchiefs and aprons sent from the body of Paul to be laid upon the sick as their point of contact for healing.

A point of contact is something you do that can cause you to release your faith, your belief system, toward God. It's like turning on a faucet to make water come out or flipping a switch to make the lights come on. It's more than just having faith because Romans 12:3 says God has given to every person *"the measure of faith."* But you must believe God's healing power is true and it's for you (Hebrews 11:1, 6). Your faith, your belief system in God's ability, must come out of you and be released toward God.

My point of contact is God's presence in my hand, which I feel from time to time, but yours can be something entirely different. I remember a friend telling me shortly after he had heard me talk about a point of contact that he knew a man who had been healed of tuberculosis while shaking the hand of his pastor at the Sunday morning service. The man had said, "When my pastor shakes my hand, that will be the moment when I believe God to heal my lungs." His healing began that very instant, for it had been his point of contact.

I have prayed for many hundreds of thousands of people since 1947. I have tried to draw strength and encouragement from those who understood my message and who used me as their instrument so that they might better release their faith toward God. Not all have been healed, but unquestionably, we have witnessed some of the greatest miracles of all times. Some of these healings have been of a nature expected by all believing Christian people. A few, however, have been outside the normal course of events. I am wholly unable to explain them, but they show God's sovereignty using a point of contact.

THE MIRACULOUS HIP SOCKET

I cannot say that this type of miracle can be had by everyone. Sometimes, even I am surprised. One time, a mother brought her child, who was on crutches, to me for prayer during one of my ministry services. She said her child had been born without a hip socket. Immediately, I told her that I felt healing, as I had seen it in my ministry, was for the recovery of a diseased part of the body and not for the restoration of a missing organ or limb. I said that in my opinion, what she was asking for would have to wait until heaven. By this time, the crowd was leaning forward, more alert than ever to the prayer line.

I frankly told the woman I did not have faith for this miracle, and I felt that I should not pray. She looked at me and said, "Brother Roberts, I don't ask you to have faith for my child. All I ask you to do is place your right hand upon him and pray. That's my point of contact. If you'll do that, I will do the believing, and God will heal my child." I remember hearing an audible gasp from the audience. Her words struck us all with such force that there was an involuntary cry from everyone. I said, "I will pray. But she will have to do the believing." I remember how it felt when I touched the place where his hip should have been. I prayed and sent them on. I am quite sure the audience believed much more than I did, and I am certain that the mother believed. The following evening when I arrived at the tent, one of my helpers met me at the car and told me the little boy had been brought back and was now being presented to the audience. I said, "Why are they doing this?" He said, "God has created his hip socket!"

It seemed incomprehensible to me; it was beyond my belief. A little later, they brought the boy to me behind the platform. He walked up to me without his crutches or any trace of a limp. The first thing I did was to place my hand over his hip where I had touched him the night before. It was no longer sunken in! The mother told me she had returned to the doctor that day, and everyone had been amazed.

I still do not have the full answer or explanation for this miracle. I believe it is an example of the kind of miracle that can happen when people have a point of contact and are able to release their faith to God. They touch the realm beyond all human understanding.

I have asked many times why I do not feel the presence of Christ in my hand all the time. I know that since this sign has come, the percentage of people being healed has increased. This gives me hope that someday, God will perform a mass miracle and an entire audience will be completely healed in an instant. I have seen this one brief time in my ministry, and I am expecting it to happen again. I have felt for several years now that we will someday see healings on this scale.

First, however, I believe we must all understand that healing is from God, and that people like me are only His instruments. We must see ourselves in this light and strive to follow God's instructions to "be like Christ and bring healing to the people as He did."

RESPONDING WITH YOUR SPIRIT

Watch and listen to a stringed musical instrument responding to the touch of human fingers. The fingers respond to what the musician is feeling inside. In the same way, your body and your mind respond or react to the force within you, the vital life force God calls your soul.

At a musical recital, I watched a young man playing the violin. I was fascinated by the remarkable sounds, the harmony, the beauty. From where I sat, it seemed like the violin was responding only to the touch of his human fingers. But I realized behind his fingers and hand was something much more important: the countless hours of practice in learning the mechanics of playing the violin and the imprint of his professor upon his spirit to understand that piece of music. Deeper still, behind it all, was the inner man or spirit translating instrument, so that presto! It felt like the beautiful music was created to calm and uplift us.

A person's mind can create and set in motion many wonders, and his body can help bring them into being. But the inner self, the spirit, is the real guiding force so that what the mind and body do—for good or for bad—is first received from the inside.

YOUR SPIRIT CAN AWAKEN

A person can awaken inwardly to the moving of the Spirit while quite young—or when quite old. Through a combination of needs I felt as a seventeen-year-old boy, my spirit awakened and directed my mind and body into repentance of my sins so that I could be born again. I prayed the sinner's prayer, "Lord, be merciful to me a sinner," and believed in my heart that God received me, and He did. It is from this beginning when I was a young man that I continually renewed myself daily in the Spirit to help me be a good disciple, or follower, of my Savior Jesus Christ.

On the stairsteps to eternity, we sometimes trip and fall back a step or two, but we can always get up and start climbing again. The important thing to me is that I am on the stairway; I am climbing and someday I'll be at the top with God forever. I will be able to go through death and enter into heaven, living forever as a whole person. The new birth started all that for me.

A person can awaken to his need for the new birth in his early or middle years, or in his mature years as my eighty-four-year-old friend did. I like to say, "It's never too late." And I always add, "But it is later than you think." Whether you're old or young, I believe that now is the time for you to decide to walk with God.

PART 2

HEALING IS MORE THAN PHYSICAL

5

DEALING WITH NEGATIVITY

Throughout my life and ministry, I've had to deal with negative situations and things that lead to negative reactions in my life. So I included this chapter of my own personal learning experiences and how I dealt with these negative reactions personally. I pray you can glean from my personal thoughts.

I believe the complex interaction between internal emotional feelings and external stresses can shape overall health.

EXPECT A NEW MIRACLE EVERY DAY

One of the most exciting times of my life occurred during our crusade in Miami, Florida. For hours, God dealt with me almost as if we were face-to-face. My entire being was quickened by His presence and He said several things to me. This is the twelfth time that I had heard God's voice.

During the prior few months, I had lived under the shadow of severe persecution. I cannot say I ever got used to it, but because of particularly unusual threats that came against me, I began to experience fear—great fear. I had already been healed of tuberculosis and my life had been spared from a gunshot just inches above my head. But this was a different kind of attack. I was not fearing for my life, but for the very existence of my ministry. An atheist group had made threats in the press, on the radio, and on television to break up our crusade on the pretext that I had laid my hands on the sick and prayed for God to heal them and this constituted practicing medicine without a license. Although they knew their argument would not stand up in court, they felt that if they succeeded in having me arrested, it would put my ministry in a bad light and elevate them in eyes of the public.

In speaking to me over the years, God has always spoken like a commander addressing a soldier—in clear, crisp terms. He said to me, "Do not fear these men. If you were put in jail, it would not hurt your ministry. I have given you a strong and solid ministry, and I Myself am with you."

ACCUSED OF SHOCKING PEOPLE

I was required by this group of atheists to stand before a judge in Miami and swear under oath that I did not have any kind of electrical device up my sleeve when I prayed for people that shocked them into healing. I was cleared by the judge, but still afraid nonetheless. But while I was trying to rest in my hotel room, God gave me a phrase that I have used every day of my life from that day on. While I was so concerned about whether the crusade would be stopped or whether they would try to arrest me, the Holy Spirit spoke to me.

"Expect a miracle," He said. "Expect a new miracle every day. If it were not possible, I would not have told you."

God told me that I was to expect a miracle—and there *was* a miracle. Later that evening while I was preaching and facing the enemy's last desperate effort to stop me from praying for the sick, I felt as if God's hand was folded around my hand, and as I reached out to the people, I felt the tide turn for victory. The atmosphere was electric with the power of the Holy Spirit. There were shouting cries of victory throughout the audience. In the altar call, hundreds came streaming down the aisles to be saved. As I began to pray for the sick, the Lord spoke to me again. I told the people, "The Holy Spirit is flooding up in me so strong tonight, I feel as if I will burst. God wants to heal you and has sent me to pray for you."

I had just gotten those words out of my mouth when a man standing within twenty feet of me began to shout and jump up and down. He had been dying of heart disease, but the Holy Spirit fell upon him. He cried out, "I am healed! I am healed!" The power of God swept over the audience in wave after wave. The ministers on the platform were crying and rejoicing as God's healing power fell through the audience.

God spoke to me again. "I am not through with your crusades yet," He told me. "You are to continue strongly and go forward in the crusades. I have given you a ministry for the needs of the people. I told you in 1947 not to be like other men, but to be like Jesus and bring healing to the people as He did. I bring this to your attention again. You are to have a healing ministry as long as you live."

All my life, I have had a love for sick people because I had been ill myself almost to the point of death. God, in His mercy, raised me up and called me to pray for the sick like Jesus did. This has been the greatest challenge I have ever known.

Then God asked me a question, "When you come up before Me, do you want to come with or without scars? Do you want to come with stars or scars?" I realized then that I had asked Him *why* too many times. He said, "My Son came to me with scars, not stars." God was trying to put things right in my mind. I knew that no matter what happened to me in the future, it would happen because I was obeying Him. I was to choose joy and never be resentful.

I was never arrested in Miami, nor were they able to stop the crusade. But something was born inside of me that has continued with me every day of my life. *I expect a miracle!* No matter what has happened, I have said to myself and to anyone who would listen that with God, we can expect a miracle. We can expect a new miracle every day!

EMOTIONS ARE PART OF OUR SOUL

I believe that all of our emotions—whether fear such as I experienced during the Miami crusade or joy when someone is healed—are part of our soul. The Bible describes our soul as our mind, our will, and our emotions. As human beings, emotions are built into our very nature; they are a part of our ability to feel, respond, or react. We are emotional beings, but there is a distinct difference between being emotional and being an emotional being. The latter suggests an acknowledgment and acceptance of our emotional nature, recognizing its significance in our lives.

Scripture reminds us of the profound connection between each aspect of our total being. Proverbs 14:30 (NIV) tells us, "*A heart at peace gives life to the body, but envy rots the bones.*" Ephesians 4:26–27 (NIV) urges us to manage our emotions wisely, saying, "*'In your anger do not sin'; Do not let the sun go down while you are still angry, and do not give the devil a foothold.*" These verses acknowledge the likelihood of negative emotions but encourage us to deal with them promptly and constructively, recognizing their potential to influence our actions.

It doesn't mean the situation changes instantly or an immediate change in anyone else who is involved. In my understanding, these verses are saying it is good for me to deal with *me* and not give the devil an opportunity to get a foothold into my personal feelings.

SAY, "GOD BLESS YOU"

I learned one way to deal with negative emotions from a dear lady named Thelma Shaw. She was the beloved wife of Judge Oras Shaw, and they were dear friends to Evelyn and me. She once told us she used the "God bless you" approach when her emotions began getting her into a *reaction* mindset. She said if another person was involved, "I would breathe a little prayer, sort of take a breath, and say *of them* to myself, 'God bless you.'" Over the years, she developed this as a *response* and at her death, when Judge Shaw invited me to say a few words, I shared this with the audience. To my surprise, people all over the church were nodding their heads, remembering this about her. Obviously, many there had been helped by this terrific Christian woman.

We had the honor of telling her story, "God bless you," and hundreds wrote of the positive impact it had made on them.

Let me tell you, I found that for me, uncontrolled or misdirected emotion can hurt other people and certainly myself most of all.

If you find yourself in a similar situation, consider Thelma's "God bless you" approach and believe that it can bless you too.

BITTERNESS

Another thing I had to deal with was holding on to bitterness. Honestly, it was easy to do, especially due to the criticism I received on a regular basis. When bitterness seemed to creep into my life, I would remind myself of the words of Paul in Hebrews 12:15: *"Lest any root of bitterness springing up trouble you, and thereby ... be defiled."*

Bitterness can spring from *a root, from something planted.*

Bitterness is a powerful emotion that can take root in our hearts if left unchecked. It was easy for me to fall into the trap of bitterness, especially in the face of criticism or mistreatment. However, Scripture warns us against allowing bitterness to take hold, as it can lead to trouble and defilement.

I used to say, "Oh, he made me so bitter." God revealed to me in this Scripture and others in the Bible that my bitterness was not forced on me by someone else. I did it. I let it happen. I had planted a seed that I was allowing to take root by permitting myself to become bitter.

One man had especially been awful to me. I fought and fought with myself, calling on God to help him and to help me. Finally, I fell upon a wonderful plan. Rather than thinking of the wrongs I felt he was doing to me, I tried to think of Christ in him, and I prayed to the Christ in him who was also in me. I actually did this several times. "O Lord," I prayed, "You are in this man, and You are in me. I call upon You; help him; help me." In one of these prayers, I felt a release in my spirit. The wrongs were still there but they didn't hurt me anymore. I felt better and better until I felt God whisper in my heart, "If you trust Me, no one can ever hurt you like that over bitterness. You can only hurt yourself by planting the seed of a bad reaction."

I use this plan often, and it worked for me because I saw all of God's children are part of Christ and part of one another. I discovered I could sow a seed and reap it back when I prayed to God through Christ who is in me. When I ask for help for the other person, it is a seed I planted that comes back multiplied like any other seed. And just as a seed planted in faith yields a bountiful harvest, so can prayer bring about healing and restoration in our lives.

RESENTMENT

When you are in the public eye, as I am, the media can say or write good stories about you, but also some unflattering ones. Of course, you eat up the good ones and hope your emotions will not get you down over the bad ones. I realize that I'm not to live by compliments in the media, but I have found that they are easier on my soul. I just can't let them control my life. Paul said we are not to think more highly of ourselves than we ought (Romans 12:3).

In the short run, it was extremely tough to keep my emotions from getting the better of me, especially when the media could be so relentless.

Several years ago, an unflattering article was written about my ministry, and the man responsible was a friend of mine. It really hurt me, and I was angry. Very angry.

I honestly tried to overcome the resentment. The resentment I had in my heart was actually worse than what this man had done to me. And every time I thought about that man, I got a sick feeling in the pit of my stomach. My attitude was hindering me in dealing with other people. Finally, I realized it wasn't that I had the anger—instead, it was that anger had me!

I began praying about it, and one day, I felt God speaking deep inside me: "Oral, write this man a letter and apologize for your feelings." I thought, "What! He should apologize to me!" But God kept telling me I had to love the man as if he'd never wronged me.

So, I sat down to write the letter. And it was hard. I told the man I'd felt bad toward him, and I asked him to forgive me for it. When I mailed the letter, I was released from the anger. I considered this act a seed of faith I was planting for my feelings to change. This was the desired result for which I planted my seed. And it happened. I felt great and was able to dismiss the whole situation from my mind.

Then lo and behold, a few days later, I received a reply from the man, saying, "I am the one who needs to apologize ..." We were reconciled, and today, we are good friends. But even if he had not replied, the resentment was released in my inner man, and I received a healing in my spirit. Again, the seed-faith prayer and the seed-faith letter I wrote had paid off for us both.

SELF-PITY

For me, the emotion that was often the most negative was self-pity. I believe we all may deal with this at some time in our lives. I have found that even seemingly tough people often seethe within because they feel they are not treated fairly. I think we have every right to feel appreciated, wanted, and loved. But sometimes it appears impossible for other people to see us as we feel they should.

Self-pity hits me worse when I have worked hard and given of myself until I am worn out in my body and maybe can't sleep well for a few nights. Many people can go home and rest until it's all over, but in ministry, we can't. The work of television, prayers for people, and ministering to individuals and large groups keeps us moving, prevents us from stopping. When I hear that someone I admire has said something negative toward me, I have to constantly fight feelings of self-pity.

Of course, my darling wife Evelyn helps me. "Now, Oral," she will say, "you're just feeling sorry for yourself. You tell others wonderful things to help them; try them on yourself." She is right, and this really snaps me to attention because self-pity can destroy all God wants us to be.

HATE

Throughout my years of ministry, I've talked to many people behind prison bars because they permitted their emotions to develop into hate until they ultimately did something violent. Every prison I have visited struck me as being filled with a hatred you could feel.

I recall speaking in a large church once where I felt a lot of hate. How could that kind of hate be in a church? Because of people who planted bad seed by misdirecting their emotions and becoming extremely negative toward each other. In that situation, while I preached, I prayed that the living Christ would speak through me, and that the congregation would *feel* His love in me and through me. Later the pastor of that church told me that something happened to his people through that sermon and especially through what they felt was God's love coming out of me toward them. I realized that the good seed I had planted in my sermon had been multiplied in blessings to the people and back to me also.

You know, for me, I discovered that what people feel coming out of you is as important as what they hear you say. This was true in my sermons, as was proven in this case.

If any human being ever had a reason to feel hate, it was Jesus. The very ones He sought to help rejected Him. Ultimately, they wanted to take His life. Being rejected and hated was no picnic even for Jesus because He was a human being. Even though He was God's Son, I hope you remember He was *Man,* an emotional being like you and me.

The thing that helps me most when thinking about and dealing with my own negative feelings and reactions is the realization that in the midst of their hate, Jesus called upon His inner man and responded from His spirit rather than from the calculating logic of His mind, which could have caused Him to hate them back.

Jesus resisted hate. He was determined not to hate. As a human being, I believe it was a battle for Him to win over Himself, just as it is for us. He won by planting seeds of His love for them.

I believe Jesus loved all people, but He loved Himself too. He knew that hate, like acid, can damage the vessel in which it is stored just as it does the object on which it is poured. I always found that hatred can cloud a person's reason. It can perhaps feel like it's punishing a person until all they think of is punishing someone else.

"How did You do it, Jesus?" I often ask. In studying His life and in observing His working in my life, I have concluded that *love* given or sown as a seed of faith is the answer—a love for God, a love for the other person, and a love for oneself. "Love your neighbor as you love yourself," Jesus said (Matthew 22:39). To me, He was saying, "Plant the *good* seed, not the bad."

I believe we all have self-worth; we all *are* somebody. God is keenly aware of His creation and values people. After all, He died for us all!

I had to come to believe that love for God, love for others, and love for myself could overcome the negative feelings and negative reactions I experienced. I believe the better we deal with negative emotions and reactions, the better we can position ourselves for a life of health, healing, and wholeness.

6

PEOPLE NEED HEALING

You may not need healing for your body. You may need healing for your soul. It could be that you need healing for your marriage, your finances, or your relationships. Perhaps you need healing for your business, or you need healing to get by from payday to payday. Or it could be a healing is needed for a loved one.

Third John 2 says, *"Beloved, I wish above all things that thou mayest prosper and be in health, even as thy soul prospereth."* It is God's highest wish for us to prosper and be in health, even as our soul prospers, and I believe that this prosperity is to be in *all things* and *in every way.*

For example, God gave me a miracle with my youngest son, Richard, who went away from me like I went away from my father when I was a teenager. Then one day a miracle happened. *It was a healing!*

Richard wasn't ill physically, but he received a healing from God in his spirit and in his soul. He used to say, "Dad, get off my back," but now he says with real conviction, "Dad, you are no longer on my back. I am by your side." And he really is. He is the featured singer on the *Oral Roberts and You* television program and host of our *Sunday Night Live* program. He is at my side in a leadership capacity as we conduct the business affairs of the ministry. He also conducts miracle services of his own all across the United States and in other countries, with outstanding miracles happening. I tell you, for me, that's the sweetest news a father can ever hear from his son or daughter! You see, this healing started *inside.*

WHAT A SURGEON SAID ABOUT A HEALING IN THE BIBLE

The miracle healing of the man with the withered hand, recorded in Mark 3:1–5, says God has the healing of your total self in mind. In this, God sees a cure or a healing differently than man does. Jesus did not focus His attention solely on the man's withered hand. He first spoke to the man himself and said, *"Stand forth." You* is implied here, meaning, "You stand forth!"

A surgeon friend of mine was talking to me about this particular miracle. He said, "Oral, as a doctor, I would have automatically turned my attention to the man's hand. This goes back to my medical training. But as I read this story, I noticed that Christ did not touch the man's crippled hand. He seemed to view it as an extension of the man's entire personality ... and within the healing of the whole person, his hand was restored."

Then my friend added a statement that I thought was tremendous. He said, "More and more, I believe medicine is moving in this direction—toward whole-person healing."

YOUR FAITH CAN MAKE YOU WHOLE

Time and time again during the ministry of Jesus, He spoke the healing word like this, "Your faith has made you whole" (Luke 17:19). The word *whole* means to keep safe and sound, to save a suffering one, to save or rescue. To me, it's well-being in your total self. This is my desire for myself and those I minister to. I encourage you to commit to being *made* a whole person. Better health and miracle-living are not only possible, but I believe they are our God-given rights!

I believe the journey to making you whole begins in your spirit, which God created in His spiritual likeness. This likeness or image is God's essence, the essence of His own being. To be born of God in your spirit today is a restoration of God's own essence or nature to yourself. You can take on this spiritual reality in your being. Through it, you can learn to respond to every situation you face by using your spirit—your inner self—then let this response flow up through your soul (your mind, will, and emotions) and body until your response is the whole-person response. You can face disease or dis-harmony as God intended—from your spirit, which is God's own way of doing it.

I've always thought that there are several all-important things to learn about God, ourselves, and our response to whatever we face in life. I believe it's important to learn about how God made you (and remakes you by giving you a new spiritual rebirth), to learn about the way God does things and trying by faith to do them as He does, and to learn that although you are flesh (human), you can respond to life first through the spiritual nature God recreates in you.

This thrills me, and I hope it thrills you too. I hope you will keep responding from your spirit for the rest of your life!

YOUR RESTORATION TO WHOLENESS IS GOD'S IDEA

There is no record in the Bible of anyone begging God to redeem or restore mankind. But *God* thought, planned, and provided for our restoration to oneness with Himself without being asked. In Genesis 3:15 (NKJV), God foreshadows this reconnection with the body of believers, saying, *"He shall bruise your head"*—He being Jesus, and *your head* being the devil's. This verse is a prophecy about the eventual victory of Christ over the forces of evil.

Although the Old Testament ends with the prophet Malachi speaking to people to repent of their sins and get right with God, the New Testament begins with the birth of a Baby and the promise of abundant life, the beginning of the promised reunification of the church.

In Matthew 1:21, we read, *"Thou shalt call his name JESUS: for he shall save his people from their sins."* And in John 10:10, we read, *"I am come that they might have life, and that they might have it more abundantly."*

Jesus is not only a Savior from sin but also a Savior of *persons.* The Greek word *sozo* means "to save" and "to heal." So, Matthew 1:21 can also mean, "You shall call His name Jesus for He shall *heal* persons. He shall *heal* them from their sins, their shortcomings, their failures, and the disharmony in their nature. He shall *heal* their bodies, their *minds—their whole beings.* He sent Jesus to give them *abundant* life."

How does Jesus do this? He begins in the Spirit. Jesus, the Man, had to be sent from His heavenly Father to be born on earth. This is why Jesus said, *"Except a man be born ... of the Spirit, he cannot enter into the kingdom of God. ... Ye must be born again"* (John 3:5, 7). He was teaching the connection between God the Father and Jesus the Son. He was connecting heaven and earth with God and His creation, mankind.

Let's get back to basics. When speaking of the spiritual rebirth in Christ, Jesus didn't say, "You must be born of the soul or of the body." He said we must be born of the Spirit! Jesus recaptured the possibility of a new birth so you can be reborn in the spiritual likeness of God. No longer must you be separated from God. No longer must your spirit be put down. But once again, your spirit can be put in charge and made the source of your total response to life. This is the new birth, your spiritual birth, that Jesus says you must have after your own natural physical birth.

I SEE THE FIGHT AS SUPERNATURAL

When Jesus came, He cared about the concerns of people. He healed all kinds of problems—sickness, poverty, soul needs, money needs, and so forth. Each time Christ approached a person, I believe it was not merely from the standpoint of his problem but from the knowledge that his whole person was in need of restoration. Because we are spiritual beings, I have always tried to deal with things spiritually first. We *may* feel a problem physically. We may feel it financially. We may feel it emotionally. But as a Christian, I believe *the problems I face have a spiritual basis* because I mainly see them as an attack of the devil.

Perhaps you can see this more clearly as you read Ephesians 6:12 (NIV), which says, *"For our struggle is not against flesh and blood, but against the rulers, against the authorities, against the powers of this dark world and against the spiritual forces of evil in the heavenly realms."* Paul, the author of this passage of Scripture, emphasizes that the true battle for believers is not merely against other people (*"flesh and blood"*) but rather against *"spiritual forces of evil."* For me, this verse underscores the spiritual dimension of the Christian life and the need for believers to be equipped with spiritual armor (Ephesians 6:13–17) to deal with challenges. It serves as a reminder to Christians that their ultimate fight is not against human adversaries but against the spiritual forces opposed to God's purposes and the advancement of His kingdom.

YOUR SPIRIT MAN

Genesis 2:7 says, *"And the* Lord *God formed man of the dust of the ground, and breathed into his nostrils the breath of life; and man became a living soul."* Man became a *living* soul—a *spiritual* being!

From the moment of creation, this Scripture declares that God meant for man's *spirit*—*not* his soul or his body—to govern his life on earth. Man's spirit is intended to hold authority over the soul and body, bringing them together into a unified, harmonized whole person. As a Christian who spent my early years rejecting God, I now believe that without God, a person is seemingly incomplete. It is God's intention to dwell *in* the individual. Similarly, a person through the spirit will live *in* God. Acts 17:28 says, *"For in him we live, and move, and have our being; as certain also of your own poets have said, For we are also his offspring."*

We see God *in* man and man *in* God in the garden of Eden when God and man walked and talked in harmony (Genesis 3:8–10). Man's life and breath and being were coordinated in this original relationship with God. God's delight was evident in His closeness to man. God said, *"It was very good"* (Genesis 1:31).

What was good to begin with in this case was man's understanding that he was a spiritual being. As long as he chose to keep that in proper focus, he would have great well-being and success. It would be miracle-living at its highest.

I believe God created us to live our whole lives by the spirit. To get God's answer for your problems, I encourage you to get into the Bible and into the *spirit*—*God's Spirit and your spirit*— looking to see how you were made and the way *God remakes you* when you repent of your sins, believe on Jesus as your personal Savior, and then experience His Holy Spirit working in your life every day.

GOD'S MATERIAL

The Tree of Knowledge of Good and Evil in the garden of Eden was beautiful to look upon; *it appealed to the senses*. But because God had made Adam and Eve as living spirits so that they would respond to life from their spirits first, He had forbidden them to eat of that tree or to live on the level of the physical and intellectual senses only. Therefore, when they ate of the forbidden fruit, the Bible says that immediately, "*they knew*" (Genesis 3:7).

In that moment, as a result of that choice, man's spirit was submerged, and he chose to live by his intellect. When the mind ascended above the spirit and took over, the spiritual part took a backseat, so to speak, to the natural or physical being and ceased to function as God intended as the source of man's response to Him and to life.

In that moment, man had the opportunity to choose to live on the level of his senses—what appeals to his sight, hearing, feeling, taste, and smell.

From that moment, mankind had the choice to manage his life and do what he wanted to do rather than exist as God had made him. In a sense, it's as though he was saying, "God, I don't need You; with my intellect, my mind, I can run my own life."

From that moment, there was a disintegration of the person-hood of man as God created him—and I believe there came a separation from God or fragmentation of his spirit, soul, and body, leading to a lack of harmony and peace. I don't believe for one minute that the mind alone can perfectly cope with the frictions of life; therefore, I believe it passes off to the body some of its limitations, frustrations, fears, and troubles.

From the moment that Adam and Eve ate from the Tree of Knowledge of Good and Evil, man was no longer God's masterpiece because now sin had marred him. But thank God, we are still

God's material! And through Jesus Christ, God's Son, we can be made whole (1 Thessalonians 5:23).

Despite this separation from God in the garden of Eden, there is hope. Jesus, through His sacrifice, has paved the way for our reconnection with God. Christ's selfless act on the cross restored the connection between our spirit and God, offering us the opportunity to live eternally in harmony with Him. Through Christ, by receiving Him as our personal Savior and Lord of our lives, we are once again connected or restored to God as His masterpiece, His cherished children. As Romans 8:13 affirms, by living through the Spirit and aligning ourselves with God's will, we can experience true life in Him.

LESSONS FROM THE POOL OF BETHESDA

Let's look at five lessons we can learn from Jesus's miracle at the pool of Bethesda in John 5:1–9:

After this there was a feast of the Jews; and Jesus went up to Jerusalem. Now there is at Jerusalem by the sheep market a pool, which is called in the Hebrew tongue Bethesda, having five porches. In these lay a great multitude of impotent folk, of blind, halt, withered, waiting for the moving of the water. For an angel went down at a certain season into the pool, and troubled the water: whosoever then first after the troubling of the water stepped in was made whole of whatsoever disease he had. And a certain man was there, which had an infirmity thirty and eight years. When Jesus saw him lie, and knew that he had been now a long time in that case, he saith unto him, Wilt thou be made whole? The impotent man answered him, Sir, I have no man, when the water is troubled, to put me into the pool: but while I am coming, another steppeth down before me. Jesus saith unto him, Rise, take up thy bed, and walk.

And immediately the man was made whole, and took up his bed, and walked: and on the same day was the sabbath.

LESSON 1: SICKNESS TAKES DIFFERENT FORMS

There were a lot of people at the pool at Bethesda in Jerusalem because they were ill in some way and believed that when the angel moved the waters, the first one to get in the pool would be healed of their ailment. I am sure it was pretty exciting to have a try at the waters that supposedly carried healing in them.

Many people today are ill in some way. Sickness takes different forms—in the body, the soul, the spirit, our relationships, or our attitude.

Not every need for healing is a physical one. As a young boy picking cotton, my arms were scarred up to my elbows, and I remember thinking, "I will never be poor again." I was so hurt by my lack that it instilled a fear in me that I struggled with well into adulthood. God had to remind me time and time again that He can supply my needs and heal my heart of the fear of not having enough.

LESSON 2: HEALING COMES FROM GOD

When it comes to believing for healing, I think understanding how to *rise up in your spirit*—the inner man that believes God and is standing upon that belief inside—may be one of the most important lessons you can learn.

This perspective can free us from a way of thinking that could fragment God's ways of healing.

French surgeon Ambroise Paré (1510–1590) often said, "I dressed the wound, but God healed him." He was acknowledging the partnership between human effort and God's divine intervention in the healing process. The Bible says in James 5:15, "*The prayer of faith shall save the sick, and the Lord shall raise him up.*"

Personally, I believe this Scripture aligns perfectly with the perspective that whichever method God uses in healing, whether the obviously miraculous or the seemingly natural, is good and acceptable—and more power to both!

LESSON 3. ALIGN YOUR WILL WITH GOD'S WORD

The story of the man at the pool of Bethesda illustrates to me how Jesus addressed not only the physical ailment but also the spirit, soul, and body of the individual.

Entrenched in the belief that his healing depended solely on the physical phenomenon of the stirred waters, the man seemingly had overlooked the deeper spiritual aspect of his condition. His encounter with Jesus brought forth a profound question: *"Do you want to get well?"* (John 5:6 NIV). This question pierced through the layers of the man's physical infirmity, prompting him to look at his entire being.

In carefully reading this story, the way I see it, Jesus, in His response, didn't only provide physical healing but initiated a transformation that began with aligning the man's will with God's intention for his life. This encounter emphasizes that true healing encompasses the spiritual, the soul, and the physical aspects of our existence. For me, it highlights to a greater degree the importance of surrendering our will to God's plan for our lives.

I believe true biblical healing starts from within, from a place of surrendering our desires, fears, and doubts to God. As I read this passage in John 5, I find this story demonstrates the need for individuals to recognize that their ultimate biblical wholeness is connected to the alignment of their own will with God's will.

4. GOD USES VARIOUS MEANS AND METHODS TO HEAL

The man at the pool of Bethesda appeared to be fixated solely on the physical manifestation of healing through the stirred waters. He didn't seem to realize the multitude of ways in which God could work in his life. When Jesus asked the man if he aligned his will with God's to be made whole, he replied, *"Sir, I have no man, when the water is troubled* [bubbling up], *to put me into the pool"* (John 5:7). He had what I call *tunnel vision,* and I believe that kind of limited perspective can perhaps hinder people from achieving better health or in seeing life as a whole.

I believe that all this man could see at the other end of his tunnel was the pool of water—and he hoped he would get in first. He had failed for thirty-eight years. His tunnel vision limited his perspective, hindering him from recognizing that God's healing power is greater than any singular method or human intervention. Similarly, we can sometimes find ourselves trapped in tunnel vision, without acknowledging all the possible resources of God's healing process.

Whenever I read the story of this man's healing, it encourages me to broaden my understanding and embrace the uniqueness of God's healing methods.

It is my hope that we learn to put all of God's delivery systems of healing and wholeness where they belong—in *Him.* We can know God and through our spirit, we can align our will with His to be made whole. We don't have to limit our thinking the way the man at the pool of Bethesda did.

By acknowledging God as the complete and total Source of healing, we can open ourselves to the possibility that God can make a way where there seems to be no way. He can bring about healing in ways we may not have even considered possible.

LESSON 5: JESUS IS CONCERNED ABOUT THE WHOLE PERSON

What is interesting about this story is that Jesus was very aware of the man's suffering body, but He began the healing process by talking to him about his condition and desires.

Matthew 9:12–13 (NIV) reinforces this by saying, "*On hearing this, Jesus said, 'It is not the healthy who need a doctor, but the sick. But go and learn what this means: "I desire mercy, not sacrifice." For I have not come to call the righteous, but sinners.*'"

At the pool at Bethesda, Jesus saw a *person* inside the body, and that inner person seemed to be lying down. Still, the man wanted his body healed. Perhaps he had not recognized that Jesus was concerned about his whole person, or that his healing could begin in his spirit. By healing this man, Jesus uplifted him. My darling wife Evelyn used to call healing *the dinner bell to salvation* for all to experience. This story is just such a dinner bell!

WHAT A PHYSICIAN TOLD ME

A physician told me recently that he believed medical and surgical help could be many times more consistent and longer lasting if doctors could get patients to understand that a positive attitude on their part will aid in their healing and recovery. In other words, I believe he meant they need faith for their healing. He said physicians use medical terms rather than theological ones because that is their training and expertise. However, this doctor believed that the healing process could possibly take on a new dimension when something happens inside the inner man of a sick person.

I shared with him the encounter Jesus had with the man at the pool. I read John 5:8 (NKJV) to him, saying, "*Jesus said to him, 'Rise, take up your bed and walk.*'" I shared how Jesus's conversation with the man seemed to begin with his spirit or inner man. I believe he was trying to encourage the man on the inside first and finally told him to do three things:

1. "*Rise.*"

2. "*Take up your bed.*"

3. "*And walk.*"

JESUS SAID, "THOU ART MADE WHOLE!"

These are cheering words to me. Jesus's words, *"Thou art made whole"* (John 5:14) convey the possibility of total wellness.

Jesus uses a making process. *"Made whole"* is what He says, but I feel like there's much involved in that, not the least of which is receiving God's delivery systems. I believe it's using our will as well as our faith, responding to prayer, and understanding how God designed our spirit to be the best responder we can have to get our soul and body moving in a biblical way toward being made whole.

PART 3

WHAT TO DO IF YOU NEED HEALING

7

MY SIX KEYS TOWARD HEALING AND WHOLENESS

I believe Jesus's highest wish is for us to prosper and have health in spirit, soul, and body.

The apostle John writes in 3 John 1:2, *"Beloved, I wish above all things that thou mayest prosper and be in health, even as thy soul prospereth."*

The story of Jesus is a story of healing and deliverance. He makes people whole in spirit, soul, and body. In the power of His pure and healthy being, He came into this world to bring people release from fears and frustrations, to set them free from spiritual and physical illnesses, and heal them in any other area that needed it in order to make them whole.

The Bible shows us that the healing Jesus brings is to make us *whole*—healthy in spirit, soul, and body, healthy in our relationships with others, our attitudes, and our way of life, all the days of our lives.

In studying God's Word, I find Jesus's desire is to deliver God's precious creation completely from all life's hurts and ills.

A LEGEND OF THE CROSS

An old legend handed down to us tells how the wooden cross on which Jesus died brought healing. The story doesn't come from Scripture, but I do like the message it conveys:

> *Helena, the mother of Constantine, while on a pilgrimage to Jerusalem, gave instructions to search for the cross of Christ. As the workmen looked through the rubbish heaps of Calvary, they found three crosses, but the inscription which was over the head of Christ was lying in a separate place. There was no clue as to which of the three crosses was the one on which our Lord died.*
>
> *Maarius, the minister of the Christian church in Jerusalem, said, "We will test the true cross." The sick were gathered together. They tried one cross, but there was no leaping of the lame nor opening of the eyes of the blind. They tried the second cross, yet there was no response. But when they tried the third cross, blind eyes were opened, deaf ears were unstopped, the lame leaped to their feet, and the sick were made whole.*

The wooden cross that stood on Calvary is gone. The Christ who hung on it is ascended and reigns from heaven. Outwardly, we see the cross no more, but Jesus the Person lives on. In Him, the lost, straying, suffering multitudes of every generation may find complete deliverance. Jesus Christ is as real today as when the multitudes saw Him with their physical eyes. He is spiritual reality—the center of the plan of redemption of humanity—spirit, soul, and body.

GOD'S ABUNDANCE OF LIFE

The Bible reveals a loving Redeemer who overshadows, surrounds, and undergirds those who place their trust in Him. With ever-active concern, He watches over us. The details of our human existence are so important to Him that He has numbered the hairs of our head (Luke 12:6–7). The sparrow cannot fall to the earth without His notice, and He clothes even the lilies of the field (Matthew 10:29; 6:28–30).

I believe your life and mine are as necessary to God's design as is every thread woven into a beautiful handmade tapestry. Not only are we responsible to God, but He is also responsible for us. The course of our lives is His business. God seeks to give us life— more abundant life (John 10:10). Jesus is life itself, according to John 14:6, and He seeks to share His life with us.

In New Testament times, when people struggling with fear, frustration, sickness, and sorrow were able to get to Jesus, they found Him full of healing and ready to set them free. It didn't make any difference who they were. With faith and expectancy in God's Word, many experienced His power to make them whole. He wanted people to have faith in God and to change their ways so they could use their faith to successfully meet life's enemies.

Mark 5:25–34 tells of a woman who went to doctor after doctor only to be told nothing could be done to cure a bleeding condition with which she had suffered for twelve years. One day, she heard of Jesus and said, *"If I may touch but his clothes, I shall be whole"* (v. 28). By this act or point of contact, which I explained earlier in chapter 4, she was able to release her faith. Jesus asked, *"Who touched my clothes?"* (v. 31). When the disciples reminded Him that the entire crowd was brushing up against Him, He knew that the woman's touch was different from everyone else's. He had felt healing power or *virtue* leave His body when she made contact with His garment (Mark 5:30). That healing power made the woman whole.

This woman had come with her need. When she touched Jesus's clothes in faith, she tapped into the healing power of Christ and was instantly healed. This is a beautiful example of God's abundance of life, which can be available to all of us.

If this sounds too good to be true, then please read and believe Jesus's words in John 10:10: *"I am come that they might have life, and that they might have it more abundantly."* Jesus is a fountain of abundant life, a life available to everyone who turns away from sin so their souls are unfettered, and their faith can be released.

Jesus rejoices over the faith that is released for liberation from sin, from the evil powers of sickness and disease, and from fear and frustration (Matthew 8:13; 15:28; Luke 8:48; 10:17–24). When we allow our faith to take hold of God's promises, His mighty power of life can surge into action on our behalf, and we are liberated. God is glorified in our faith, which brings His answer to our prayers.

SIX KEYS TOWARD HEALING

Now, with these thoughts in mind, I urge you to consider these six keys to healing that have shaped my life and ministry. I believe they can help you understand your biblical rights regarding healing:

1. Believe that it is God's will to heal you and make you a whole person.

Many Christians recognize that God has healing power. Simple acceptance of this truth is wonderful ... but knowing or believing is not the same thing as standing in faith for miracles. I believe we must have personal, active faith in God for our personal healing.

If God has ever healed one person, He can heal two; if He heals two, He can heal four; if four, then eight, and so on. He can heal all who will believe. Otherwise, He would have healing compassion for one and not another. But *"there is no respect of persons with God"* (Romans 2:11), meaning that He does not show partiality or favoritism. Healing comes about because of faith, not favoritism.

I love God because He first loved me (1 John 4:19). I love Him because He loves me *and* my family *and* my friends *and* all other people. I say this because He healed me of tuberculosis and gave me wonderful health in my entire being, which I now enjoy through His love. But should He love only me, I would be disappointed, for then if my child or a friend contracted tuberculosis, it is likely (on that basis) that He would not heal the person.

It is my sincere belief that Christ's death on the cross was for all people everywhere and in all generations. The apostle Peter writes of Jesus, *"Who his own self bare our sins in his own body on the tree, that we, being dead to sins, should live unto righteousness: by whose stripes ye were healed"* (1 Peter 2:24). More than seven hundred years before the crucifixion, the prophet Isaiah had known that Christ would be the Savior and Healer. He prophesies, *"But he was wounded for our transgressions, he was bruised for our iniquities: the chastisement of our peace was upon him; and with his stripes we are healed"* (Isaiah 53:5).

The apostle Matthew tells the story of Jesus as the Great Physician, and he says that Jesus's healing power is a fulfillment of Scripture. Referring to Isaiah 53:4, Matthew writes, *"They brought unto him many that were possessed with devils: and he cast out the spirits with his word, and healed all that were sick: that it might be fulfilled which was spoken by [Isaiah] the prophet, saying, Himself took our infirmities, and bare our sicknesses"* (Matthew 8:16–17).

108 *Oral Roberts on Healing*

When Jesus healed the people of their sicknesses—in their spirit, in their soul, and in their bodies—He was freeing them from the oppression of the devil. Peter makes this clear in Acts 10:38, when he says, that God *"anointed Jesus of Nazareth with the Holy Ghost and with power: who went about doing good, and healing all that were oppressed of the devil; for God was with him."*

Sickness is not numbered among the blessings of the gospel but is counted an enemy of human life. Jesus Christ healed the people, taking from them the heavy, oppressive hand of disease, giving them life and strength. He explained that *"the Son of man is not come to destroy men's lives, but to save them"* (Luke 9:56). This inspires those of us who have received healing to share all we know with others who need healing.

God looks upon sickness as:

+ The oppression of the devil (Acts 10:38).

+ The captivity of Satan (Job 42:10) as a part of the curse of the law (Galatians 3:13; Deuteronomy 28:15, 20, 22–29, 58–61, 65, 66).

+ Something He Himself took and bore on the cross (Matthew 8:17).

+ Something to be healed and destroyed by faith and prayer and special gifts (Mark 16:17,18; James 5:15; 1 Corinthians 12:6–11).

Every act, every movement, every work of the Master was directed toward making people whole and free. When the centurion rushed to Jesus and implored His mercy to heal his suffering and dying servant, Jesus replied, *"I will come and heal him"* (Matthew 8:7). And He did!

When the woman with the issue of blood touched the hem of His garment by faith, healing went out of Jesus and made her whole (Matthew 9:20–22; Luke 8:43–48).

When the ruler cried that his daughter was at the point of death, but if Jesus would only come and lay His hands upon her, she would not die but live, Jesus went with him and raised the child (who by this time had died) to life (Mark 5:22–24, 35–42).

When blind Bartimaeus shouted, *"Jesus, thou son of David, have mercy on me"* (Mark 10:47), Jesus stopped the crowds, had the beggar brought to Him, and restored his sight, saying, *"Go thy way; thy faith hath made thee whole"* (v. 52).

These healing miracles help paint the portrait of the Great Physician. He was either on His way to heal, He was delivering the captive, or He had just left and the one who had been sick or oppressed was up and rejoicing in abundant life.

2. Remember that healing from God begins in the inner being.

You reach God and He reaches you through your soul (mind, will, and emotions). When God breathed the breath of life into man, he *"became a living soul"* (Genesis 2:7). Jesus declares, *"God is a Spirit: and they that worship him must worship him in spirit and in truth"* (John 4:24).

The Bible teaches that our soul governs our physical life and passes off to the body and mind its illnesses, its distresses, and its troubles. As the strings of an instrument respond to the touch of human fingers, our bodies respond to the impressions of our souls.

I have prayed for people with all sorts of ailments. When someone is out of tune or harmony with God, my prayer is that they reconnect with God by refocusing the soul on the things of God.

First John 3:19–24 (NKJV) says:

By this we know that we are of the truth, and shall assure our hearts before Him. For if our heart condemns us, God is greater than our heart, and knows all things. Beloved, if our heart does not condemn us, we have confidence toward God. And whatever we ask we receive from Him, because we keep His commandments and do those things that are pleasing in His sight. And this is His commandment: that we should believe on the name of His Son Jesus Christ and love one another, as He gave us commandment. Now he who keeps His commandments abides in Him, and He in him. And by this we know that He abides in us, by the Spirit whom He has given us.

I believe many struggles begin within. And the exciting thing is that Scripture says if our heart does not condemn us, then we have confidence toward God (1 John 3:21). This *"confidence toward God"* is faith. Faith is your belief system. And Romans 12:3 says that God has given to every person the measure of faith.

The question presents itself, "Do people have faith, whether they are right with God or not?" The answer is yes.

Everybody has faith, for *"God has dealt to each one a measure of faith"* (Romans 12:3 NKJV). Without the power of active faith, the soul can be, in a sense, on its own (without God's connection) and left with the difficulty of trying to figure out the grueling grind of life. The body and mind, keenly responsive to the soul, can now be left feeling the impact of the soul's fears and weaknesses and fall prey to many ills.

I believe it adds up to this: You must get right with God so God can put things right in you. God can heal both your inner and outer being. And since the Bible indicates faith to be our method of belief, what are you believing? Are you believing that you will see the goodness of God in the land of the living? Or are you putting your attention on fear, worry, and doubt—inhibiting your faith from being used the way that God intended, for His glory and your benefit (Psalm 27:13).

"Except a man be born again, he cannot see the kingdom of God" (John 3:3). The new birth is a transforming spiritual experience (2 Corinthians 5:17). Condemnation is lifted. As Romans 8:1 says, *"There is therefore now no condemnation to them which are in Christ Jesus, who walk not after the flesh, but after the Spirit."*

When a person is born again by the Spirit of God, it means a change of attitudes, a change of habits, and a change in daily living. To *"walk not after the flesh"* refers to the unselfish living of the person in Christ. I encourage you to let God into your soul and open your entire being to His healing power.

3. Use a point of contact for the release of your faith.

God is a spirit and sometimes we can be confused because He is not directly before us in a human body. We cannot see Him with the human eye, nor can we take a trip to heaven and present our case as we would go to our doctor's office and talk to our physician.

How, then, can we reach God?

I believe establishing a point of contact is key.

A point of contact is the means of sending your faith, your belief system in God, directly to Him. It is something tangible, something you do, and when you do it, you release—or put into action—your faith toward God. You may recall that in chapter 4, I explained how God told me I would feel His presence in my right hand as a point of contact with people.

Faith is the meeting ground between your limited self and your limitless God. A point of contact helps you to release your faith. Establishing a point of contact is like stepping on the gas pedal of your car—you expect something to happen.

A Roman centurion in the Bible had a point of contact when he came to Jesus about his servant who was grievously tormented. This Roman soldier said to Jesus, "*Lord, I am not worthy that thou shouldest come under my roof: but speak the word only, and my servant shall be healed*" (Matthew 8:8). Notice the centurion said, "Speak the word." He went on to say, "*For I am a man under authority, having soldiers under me: and I say to this man, Go, and he goeth; and to another, Come, and he cometh; and to my servant, Do this, and he doeth it*" (v. 9).

This Roman soldier is saying that he recognizes authority and is obedient to it. He knew that his master, Caesar, did not have to be present for his commands to be carried out, because the power and authority of the empire were vested in Caesar. This power was delegated to the emperor's soldiers; therefore, when the centurion would give an order to the soldiers under him, they would obey without question.

"Now," the Roman centurion was essentially saying to Jesus, "You have authority over my servant's affliction. You don't need to come to my house. I am not worthy of such an honor. Just say *the word* that my servant shall live, and I will believe it, returning home with assurance that he is well."

This is an example of living faith—unquestioning, unfaltering, simple, childlike faith that believes God is honest and true and sends His power to accomplish what faith asks.

The Lord answered simply, "*Go thy way; and as thou hast believed, so be it done unto thee*" (Matthew 8:13). The verse goes on to say that the servant "*was healed in the selfsame hour.*"

The centurion's point of contact was the *spoken word of Jesus*, who has all power in heaven and in earth over human hurts, ills, and suffering. The moment Jesus spoke, the centurion released his faith and his servant was made whole. I believe the release of faith is the master key to healing.

I see the point of contact as what *sets the time* to deliberately connect with God. The centurion's time for the healing of his servant was to be the very moment that Jesus spoke.

Remember that the woman with the issue of blood also used a point of contact, which helped her set the time for healing. She said, "*If I may touch but his clothes, I shall be whole*" (Mark 5:28). The act of touching His clothes helped her release her faith, and her faith made her whole. I believe this is why God gives us a point of contact.

The book of Acts tells that handkerchiefs or aprons were sent from the body of the apostle Paul to those who were sick and demon-possessed, and through these faith cloths, healings were manifest (Acts 19:12). These cloths became points of contact and when placed upon the bodies of the sick and afflicted, these individuals released their faith and were set free. The important part about a point of contact is that it can be a tangible means that encourages people to release their faith and believe the Scripture that they can be healed.

Jesus is not physically present on earth today with His garments, nor is Paul with his blessed cloths. But God has not left Himself without human instruments to deliver this generation.

We read in Hebrews 6:1–3 that the laying on of hands is a Christian doctrine. I believe that one of the highest expressions of the Christian faith is when believers in Jesus put their hands on a person in prayer. When we lay hands on people, we are stepping out of our place of comfort and identifying with distressed and suffering people, allowing the anointing of the Lord to move on someone else's behalf. To me, we are having faith with them for their healing and believing for it with them. This is one reason I lay my hands on the people when I minister to them in prayer. It's not about my hands any more than it is about a prayer cloth or anointing oil. When I do these things, I am calling on the anointing and power of God—the tangible presence of the spirit of God to work through me or through any point of contact as we release our faith.

It's not about *man* healing; it's about God's anointing moving on a person to bring healing to the sick. I know that my hands cannot heal. Only God can do that. But my hands serve as a point of contact for releasing my faith and also their faith for people to be healed. When I touch someone with my hands in prayer, my heart and my compassion seem to flow through my hands. All my faith, all my feeling, and all the intensity of my belief in God are poured out in this contact and I ask God for everything He desires to do in a particular moment seems to be expressed through the laying on of hands.

Jesus said of those who believed, *"They shall lay hands on the sick, and they shall recover"* (Mark 16:18).

James 5:14–15 teaches:

> *Is any sick among you? Let him call for the elders of the church; and let them pray over him, anointing him with oil in the name of the Lord: and the prayer of faith shall save the sick.*

Elders are the spiritual leaders in the church—ministers such as pastors, evangelists, teachers, and laypeople too. The anointing oil is a symbol of the Holy Spirit. There is no healing in the oil itself, but it is also a point of contact to help people release their faith.

Keep in mind, the laying on of hands was my point of contact when I was healed in 1935, where the prayer of faith was made to God on my behalf.

I had been bedfast for five months with tuberculosis in both lungs. As I was being taken to the meeting on a mattress in the backseat of a car in this condition, I was led to use the anointing oil and the laying on of hands as a point of contact. Deep in my heart, I was believing in God for deliverance; and I told the Lord that when the evangelist anointed me and laid his hands on my head, *then* would I believe the work was done.

At that time, I had never heard of using a point of contact to release my faith to God. I had been taught that God uses the laying on of hands in prayer for the healing of the sick, but no one had told me to make that my point of contact and send my faith to God the moment hands were laid on me. But that's exactly what I did, and I can testify to its reality and effectiveness.

The prayer line was long. Midnight came, and I was still waiting. Although I was suffering, I did not become discouraged or angry at having to be the last person prayed for. Trembling with anticipation, I waited for the evangelist to anoint me and touch me with his hands. At last, my time came.

I was helped to my feet. I watched every move the evangelist made. Above all, I was watching for him to place his hands on my head. Then the anointing oil touched my forehead. His hands were upon me, and at that instant, I sent my faith to God. The deepest desires and emotions of my hungry spirit pushed outward toward God. I believed God! I found myself thanking Him for deliverance. Every ache and pain disappeared. Glory rushed into my soul. I was tingling from head to toe with new life. And then, for several minutes, I was lost in the joy of divine deliverance. I opened my eyes a little later, astonished to realize that I was leaping and shouting and running on the long platform. I was healed through faith in God!

Because of the evidence I experienced in my own life, I urge you to release *your* faith. Hold nothing back. Pour all of your faith into the act of believing for God to make you whole.

4. Release your faith—now.

So many times, I have realized the need to tell someone, "Believe *now.*" On the other hand, many people, if asked when they expect to get healed, will reply, "When God is ready, I am." I have always believed that God has been ready all the time and that the next move is up to the person. Others reply, "I'm expecting God to heal me any time." This statement seems to have a certain amount of value, but I believe that there is a definite time when faith works. God says, *"Now is the day of salvation"* (2 Corinthians 6:2), meaning the time for salvation, including deliverance from sickness and disease.

The Bible says God wants to heal you. The best time is when God is ready, and as 2 Corinthians 6:2 says, "He is ready now."

The woman with the issue of blood set a time for her healing—when she touched Jesus's garment. The centurion set a time for his servant's deliverance—when Jesus spoke the word. The ruler of the synagogue set a time for Jesus to raise his daughter from the dead when he said to Him, *"Come and lay thy hand upon her, and she shall live"* (Matthew 9:18). Each of these individuals expected deliverance at the moment the Lord did what they asked Him to do. I have always believed that God responds and works on our behalf when we believe and set the time. This is a glorious privilege and matchless opportunity.

I want to encourage you to believe God for deliverance this very minute. If faith has risen in your heart, release it to Him. Believe God now. I believe the secret of deliverance is obedience.

5. Close the case for victory.

When the conditions set forth in Scripture have been met and you feel God's healing power surge through your body in answer to the faith prayer, then close the case. Look to God and believe Him every step of the way. Consider not talking about the affliction except when God especially impresses you to give your testimony. In my personal healing, I felt led to dwell more on His mighty power of deliverance than on what the devil afflicted me with and how I suffered. I encourage you to consider this as the Lord leads you, and guard your word so that you can continuously walk out your victory with glorious faith.

6. Join yourself to companions of faith.

I know how important it was for me to have encouragement and to be able to live in an atmosphere of faith after having been healed.

If you remember, just a few days after I had been healed from tuberculosis, I felt extremely weak in my body. My mother, a devout woman of faith, sensed my discouragement and said, "Son, you were sick a long time, and you were bedfast for more than five months when God healed you. You will have to exercise and do some work to get your strength back. The Lord knows all about it, Son. You just keep your faith in Him." I say she *saved* my healing.

I have often wondered what would have happened to me had my mother and father not provided an atmosphere of faith during those early days of my healing. I have asked myself these questions: What if I had associated with a group that was unfriendly toward healing and those who had been healed? What would I have done in a moment of weakness and despondency if people had failed to encourage me or if they had ridiculed me? Having been healed by a miracle, how could I have received help from a group that denied the possibility and reality of the miracle of healing God had done in me through faith in Him? How would I have survived had I listened to people who ridiculed those who had prayed for me?

In my experience, I found only one answer to this problem. After receiving deliverance by faith in God, whenever possible, I tried to associate with Christians who practiced positive faith in God and created an atmosphere of God's love in which to live.

8

TALKING WITH GOD ABOUT
YOUR HEALING

A woman in the Bible was faced with a vexing problem. We find her story in Matthew 15:22–28:

> *And, behold, a woman of Canaan came out of the same coasts, and cried unto him, saying, Have mercy on me, O Lord, thou son of David; my daughter is grievously vexed with a devil. But he answered her not a word. And his disciples came and besought him, saying, Send her away; for she crieth after us. But he answered and said, I am not sent but unto the lost sheep of the house of Israel. Then came she and worshipped him, saying, Lord, help me. But he answered and said, It is not meet to take the children's bread, and to cast it to dogs. And she said, Truth, Lord: yet the dogs eat of the crumbs which fall from their masters' table. Then Jesus answered and said unto*

her, O woman, great is thy faith: be it unto thee even as thou wilt. And her daughter was made whole from that very hour.

When there was absolutely no hope for her little girl to be restored to normal living, she did the one thing each of us can do. She approached Jesus with her problem and secured deliverance, but not before she was turned down three times! And every refusal was an answer. God's *no* is just as much an answer as His *yes*. She finally understood Jesus's answers and realized why He had turned her down. Then she faced herself and saw that her attitude and approach were misguided. She saw that she could not remake God, but He could remake her. She could not get Him to agree to her way, which would bring failure, but she could accept His way and secure the very thing she wanted most.

The fourth time she asked Jesus to heal her child, He healed her that very hour because this was according to His will and His word for her life (Matthew 15:28).

PUT YOURSELF IN HER SITUATION

Imagine yourself as this woman in the Scripture, taking a trip to heaven today and bringing your case before God in person. When you arrive at the gate, you meet the apostle Peter and ask, "Peter, do you suppose He will receive me and heal my child?"

Peter replies, "Now don't you worry. He will receive you. I have never known Him to turn anyone away. You go right on in and tell Him your need."

The next one you meet is Paul. You say, "Oh, Paul, I am so glad to see you! I am going in to see God. Do you think He will grant my petition?"

Paul answers, "I was the chief of sinners, and He heard my prayer. The least of the apostles, and He gave me an answer. I am sure He will not turn you away."

Later you talk with the apostle John, and he assures you that you will be given every consideration by the Lord.

Then they let you in, and you find yourself standing before the Savior.

You say, "Oh, Master, my little child is possessed with demon spirits, and I have come to You, for You alone can help me. Heal her, Lord, please."

Jesus is silent. He doesn't speak even so much as one word.

You turn and stumble out. "Oh, John, He didn't answer me even one word. Why, oh, why?"

"Now, don't be upset. Go right back in and repeat your request," says John.

The second time you stand there, the Lord replies, "I cannot help people like you."

Once more you leave, this time badly broken. You meet Paul again. "Oh, great apostle, you told me He helped you and would not turn me away. But He has just said that my kind is not acceptable to Him."

Paul answers, "Didn't you wait for Him to explain what He meant by that? You didn't leave before He finished, did you? You did, I can see that. You see, God may have a better way than yours if you will only give Him a chance to show you."

The third time you stand before the Savior and plead your cause, He says, "It is not proper to give the children's bread to dogs." This is the last straw. You can take no more. Out you go. Running up to Peter, you burst into tears and say, "He called me a dog and implied that I wasn't worthy. I'll never try again."

Then Peter takes hold of you and says very gently, "Woman, all that Jesus said to you was an answer."

"Why, He insulted me!"

"No, Jesus doesn't insult anyone."

"Well, why did He say such hard things to me?"

"Whatever He said to you, He had a reason for saying it."

"You mean He did not mean to humiliate me?"

"I can assure you that what He said was intended to reveal your attitude, to help you see that the changing of your inner self often comes before a miracle of healing."

"But I want my child healed."

"I know, but the Master wants not only to heal your child but also to do something in you."

"Do you suppose . . . ? Why, I suppose you are right, Peter. The first time I came before Him, He showed no sign of recognition. Maybe that was because I wasn't in harmony with Him and wasn't seeking to be. The next time, He said He couldn't help people like me. I felt I was as good as anybody else, but now I see I showed a very bad attitude. And now He says I am a dog! Now I remember that's a word used by the children of Israel for gentiles who do not care about God. Peter! Peter! I see it all now. He wasn't refusing me, but only trying to get me into the right condition to answer my prayer. I am going back, and this time I will know how to pray!"

This time before the Lord you say, "Truth, Lord. All You say about me is true. My life is not in harmony with Your life. But, Master, even the dogs eat of the crumbs that fall from their master's table. I believe even a tiny crumb of Your healing power can heal my daughter, Please give me a crumb, Lord."

He reaches out His hands, saying, *"O woman, great is thy faith: be it unto thee even as thou wilt"* (Matthew 15:28).

This is the story of a person coming to see Christ for who He is, seeing themselves for who they are, and seeking to change their attitude and way of life. It is also exercising their will and faith toward God.

There are so many people who hear *no* from God when they pray to Him, all because they refuse to let God truly change them. They want God on their own terms ... or not at all. Consequently, they have reached a dead end; they are stymied and frustrated. Confusion troubles them, and they have turned away from God, ceasing even to pray anymore.

I want to share with you what I believe is a way out of this kind of dilemma, a royal roadway to the place where a person can meet Christ and learn His way and follow it in life.

Here is what I believe you can do when in your prayer to God, you do not sense He is even interested in your situation.

WHEN GOD SEEMS DISINTERESTED

Suppose you pray and apparently there is no word, no response whatever from God. You can't feel any assurance, any hope that your prayer has been heard. There is no tangible evidence of the answer. Does this mean that God answers prayer indiscriminately?

God has given us an example of this in Luke 18:1–8. Jesus told the story of a widow who was unjustly treated and went to a judge to obtain justice. Imagine with me that the conversation went something like this:

The judge listened impatiently to her story and said, "Come back later."

On her next visit, he was even less courteous and brushed her off again. When she thought it over, she decided that her chances of receiving fair treatment from the unjust judge were slim—that is, unless she could provoke him to act on her behalf. She went again and stood before him.

She said, "Judge, I insist on your taking immediate action!"

"Woman," he replied, "there has been a delay in your case. I am very sorry."

Once again, she said, "Judge, I am not leaving until you take action on my behalf."

The judge summoned his secretary, but the woman would not relent.

"I am staying right here until you help me," she said.

He looked at her and saw that she meant it—and this is important. Because he saw he could not put her off any longer, he said, "Oh, all right. If it will stop you from annoying me, I will do what you say."

In this story, the unjust judge avenged the woman of her adversaries, not because he was in agreement with her cause, but because she provoked him to action by her unrelenting demands. After Jesus told this story, He said, "*And shall not God avenge his own elect, which cry day and night unto him, though he bear long with them? I tell you that he will avenge them speedily*" (Luke 18:7–8).

God is for us. If the unjust judge would help a woman only because of her insistence, how much more will God, who is in harmony with our cause, help those who come to Him with determination and faith?

In other words, when you pray to God, if you have any thought of giving up before the answer comes, I encourage you: Don't give up and keep believing until your prayer is answered.

WHAT TO DO WHEN GOD SAYS NO

Think back to the woman in Matthew 15:22–28, who approached Jesus to ask Him to heal her demon-possessed daughter. When Jesus told this woman that He was not sent to her people, but to *"the lost sheep of the house of Israel"* (v. 24), He was saying no to her prayer, but not necessarily no to her. Before it was over, even though He had said no, He gave her what she wanted— healing for her child.

I believe that when God's answer starts out with *no*, it's because He has a better way.

His *no* doesn't mean we are completely cut off from what we ask Him to do, but that we have an opportunity to examine ourselves and discover if we really want healing on God's terms or only on our own.

Sometimes when God doesn't heal right away it is because He has a greater miracle planned that serves a larger purpose. This is found in the story of Lazarus, brother to Mary and Martha, in John 11:1–45.

When Lazarus became very sick, his sisters sent for Jesus. After Jesus heard the news, He said, *"This sickness is not unto death, but for the glory of God, that the Son of God might be glorified thereby"* (vv. 3–4). Jesus stayed where He was for two days and did not return until Lazarus had been dead and buried for four days (John 11:6, 17).

So, Jesus said *no*. Yet it is recorded that He loved Martha, her sister, and Lazarus (John 11:3, 5). When Jesus had said that Lazarus's sickness was to glorify God in verse 4, He intended to raise Lazarus from the dead! Raising him from the dead would glorify God more than healing him would. When Jesus said no, He had a better way because after Lazarus had been called forth from the grave, many Jews believed in Him (John 11:45; 12:11).

Don't be afraid to trust God, for He knows what He is doing and knows best how to bless and guide us.

There may have been times in your life when you wondered where God was because you didn't see the outcome to your prayers that you desired. But I want to encourage you to continue expecting miracles. I have always relied on 1 Corinthians 13:12, *"For now we see through a glass, darkly; but then face to face: now I know in part; but then shall I know even as also I am known."* Even if you don't see your healing miracle the way you thought it would be, I encourage you to believe that God is still good and we can trust Him. We don't have to understand to know that God is still sovereign. For me, this is where hope and trust come in. I have to trust in the goodness of God and believe that He is still God in every situation.

WHAT IT MEANS WHEN GOD SAYS WAIT

When God says *wait,* it could mean that His will or purpose is involved in a special way. In other words, it may be more important to wait a little while for the working out of certain details in your life, for certain changes to come to pass, than to answer you instantly. This is sometimes true in healing. In some cases, God heals instantly, but where a higher or different purpose is involved, He says *wait.* When His will has been worked out, then the healing can take place.

As you have just read, when Jesus told Mary and Martha to wait, His will was to perform a greater miracle so that many more would believe in Him. This way, He was able to accomplish more by the delay than would have been accomplished through a quick or instant healing.

WHEN THE DEVIL INTERFERES

However, there may be an enforced wait that God has not caused.

When Daniel prayed to God for His blessing, the devil inter-fered, and Daniel had to wait twenty-one complete days for the answer. This was not because God would not respond, or that He said *no* or *wait*, but because the kingdom of Satan, the devil, was directly opposing the answer to prayer (Daniel 10:13).

I believe it happened in this manner:

The devil has authority as the *"prince of the power of the air"* (Ephesians 2:2), and he has headquarters between this earth and heaven where God's throne is in the spiritual realm. Daniel prayed in Babylon and the prayer was received in heaven. God dispatched the answer through regular channels. The demon hordes of Satan kept the answer bottled up for twenty days. Daniel continued to believe, refusing to give up. Although he could not understand the seeming delay, he would not quit praying. On the twenty-first day, God told the mighty angel Michael to take the answer through the enemy lines to His beloved servant.

Michael stormed the devil's fort, pushed through the demon guards, lifted the gates off Satan's inner sanctum, reached in and got the answer to Daniel's prayer, and kept right on going. The angel who had been sent to deliver God's answer to Daniel explained, *"O Daniel, a man greatly beloved. … From the first day … thy words were heard … But the prince of the kingdom of Persia withstood me one and twenty days"* (Daniel 10:11–13).

If you pray in all sincerity and faithfulness, according to God's will, and the answer will not come through, I believe the devil has thrown up a blockade. Hold on. God can get the answer through even if He has to put His mighty angels on the case. They can get the answer through to you.

HEALING IS THE CHILDREN'S BREAD

Think once again of the woman in Matthew 15:22–28 who had to wait for her answer. Remember, she came to ask Christ to heal her demon-possessed child. Jesus replied that she was asking for the children's bread, which He would not give to her because she was unclean, not right with God. He told the woman, *"It is not* [right] *to take the children's bread, and to cast it to dogs"* (v. 26).

Healing is the children's bread. This is why Jesus was so careful to lead this woman, to probe her soul, to work a change in her life, to get her into the attitude of humility, love, and faith.

Jesus indicates that healing is the heritage of His children. Thank God, it is! This is one of the most amazing revelations Jesus ever made. God Himself says in Exodus 15:26, *"I am the* LORD *that healeth thee."* And David writes in Psalm 103:3 that God *"forgiveth all thine iniquities"* and *"healeth all thy diseases."* Each one of us has a perfect right to God and just as He can forgive all of our sins, He can heal all of our diseases.

God not only wanted the daughter set free, He wanted the mother to be set free also. When the woman in Matthew 15 saw the truth of Christ's statements, she admitted she was not in harmony with God. She humbled her spirit and acknowledged that she needed His saving power. Remember that in response to Jesus's comment about giving the children's bread to dogs, she said, *"Yet the dogs eat of the crumbs which fall from their masters' table"* (v. 27). In other words, she was not asking for a piece of bread, just a crumb. Perhaps she asked for only a healing crumb because she felt unworthy to sit with the children. It's almost like she was saying, "Please just pitch it under the table, Lord," yet with faith, determination, and humble devotion.

Jesus was thrilled at what she said and immediately healed the woman's daughter, saying, *"O woman, great is thy faith: be it unto thee even as thou wilt"* (Matthew 15:28). The verse goes on to say, *"And her daughter was made whole from that very hour."* This woman was willing to change her attitude, humbly come before Jesus in sincere worship, and believe Him. Her faith put Jesus to work on her behalf.

Faith is always rewarded. For me, the key to receiving the things we need is our faith in God (Hebrews 11:1, 6).

But I believe He can do all things and do them well. He wants to give us more than physical healing; He wants to make us what we ought to be. He wants us to bring our whole person into harmony with Him.

When prayer is backed up by the right attitude and a willingness to change, I believe we can approach Christ, be heard, and receive according to God's will and His Word. In His way, in His timing, He answers prayer.

Let us contend together; state your case, that you may be acquitted.   (Isaiah 43:26 NKJV)

9

FIVE WAYS YOU CAN USE YOUR FAITH FOR HEALING

The story on which this chapter is based centers around General Naaman of Syria (2 Kings 5:1–15). Naaman was commander in chief of Syria's expeditionary forces and had been hailed as a national hero because of his outstanding military successes.

The general's personal physician must have been shocked when he realized his chief had contracted the disease of leprosy, which was a common condition in those days.

Across the nation, I can imagine the cry that must have gone up, "General Naaman is a leper! Our beloved leader is a leper!"

Leprosy meant living death—slow, torturous, isolated suffering.

Naaman had made a victorious march across the Bible land of Israel and had taken a girl captive to be a servant to his wife. This girl was familiar with God and His prophets and knew healing power flowed through them. Seeing that the general was a leper, she said, *"Would God my lord were with the prophet that is in Samaria [Israel]! for he would recover him of his leprosy"* (2 Kings 5:3).

Naaman was grateful for this hope, believed the girl's message, and made preparations to leave for Israel.

In the ancient story of Naaman's miraculous healing through his faith in God and throughout the New Testament, we see five ways we can use our faith for healing today.

RECOGNIZE SICKNESS AND DISEASE AS THE OPPRESSION OF THE DEVIL

This rule of faith is made plain to us by Simon Peter, one of Jesus's twelve apostles. He was well aware of the Savior's love for suffering humanity. After Christ's resurrection, Peter was preaching to the soldiers in the house of Cornelius in Caesarea. He said, *"God anointed Jesus of Nazareth with the Holy Ghost and with power: who went about doing good, and healing all that were oppressed of the devil; for God was with him"* (Acts 10:38).

Jesus *"went about doing good"* and *"healing all that were oppressed"* by the devil; this is Peter's summation of the Lord's ministry.

Disease is a foul and inhuman thing and is not numbered among the blessings of life. Jesus Christ came against it in the power of His pure and healthy humanity, laying His healing hands upon the sick and tormented, *"healing every sickness and every disease among the people"* (Matthew 9:35). People touched Him too. The Bible states, *"As many as touched him were made whole"* (Mark 6:56).

Satan is a destroyer of human life, while Jesus is a destroyer of the oppressions (human afflictions) of the devil.

The writers of the four Gospels—Matthew, Mark, Luke, and John—tell the story of Jesus and His healing power. All of them tell how Jesus found the people oppressed with all manner of sickness, all manner of disease, and the unusual manifestations of demons. They tell how He healed their sick (Matthew 4:23; 14:14; Mark 1:29–34; Luke 4:33–36; 18:35–43; John 4:46–53). They teach us that compassion flowed through Him like the water of a pure mountain stream and became healing power for all who would believe (Matthew 14:14; Mark 1:40–42; Luke 7:12–15). The healing power of Jesus is God's antidote for sickness and is available to all who place their faith in Him.

According to the Bible, the Savior did not turn away any person who had faith. He simply looked for faith; wherever He found it, He healed the sick. One of His favorite expressions was, *"As thou hast believed, so be it done unto thee"* (Matthew 8:13).

He healed the blind, the deaf, the demon possessed, the feverish, the brokenhearted, and many others. The apostle Peter would have witnessed many healing miracles Jesus did, and later, in writing of Jesus, he declares, *"by whose stripes ye were healed"* (1 Peter 2:24).

Jesus imparted healing power to His followers (Matthew 10:1–8; Luke 10:1–9; John 14:12–14), and many of them saw God's power deliver people from sickness and disease in remarkable ways. In Acts 5:15, we read that those on whom Peter's shadow fell were healed. He never had to lay hands on them. This was after the day of Pentecost (Acts 1:8; 2:1–4). Similarly, Stephen and Philip, laymen of the early church, ministered healing to many people through faith (Acts 6:8; 8:6–7).

Paul describes the nine gifts of the Holy Spirit in 1 Corinthians 12. These include the gifts of healing, faith, discerning of spirits, and miracles (vv. 9–10). These gifts are mighty in healing the sick and casting out demons. They are additional gifts to go along with faith and can help in bringing deliverance.

Gifts from God can be used in helping the deliverance of others as God directs.

This, then, is our God: loving, tender, compassionate, and full of healing power. Satan is an oppressor; Christ is the Life Saver (John 10:10). Just as Satan is the source of torment, God is the source of life. Christ's healing ability for people can be found everywhere faith is found as people are looking to Him for health, peace, and happiness.

Remember, the Bible pictures Jesus as coming into a world full of sickness and demon possession. When certain religious leaders would not work with Him, He went alone, but He was not alone *"for God was with him"* (Acts 10:38). He chose everyday individuals to be His partners, and He transmitted His healing power through them.

He had glorious success in healing the souls and bodies of the multitudes. He never said to one, "It is *not* My will to heal you," and to another, "It *is* My will to heal you," but as God instructed, He healed those who were oppressed by the devil and who would believe.

Only once do we read in the Bible that Jesus was powerless to heal, but there was a reason for this. The people of Nazareth were His acquaintances, and they were skeptical of Him and His ministry. They looked upon the accounts of His wonders with scorn, and when He came to preach to them, they met Him with cold unbelief. The gospel writers did not omit what happened in Jesus's hometown but recorded it in a terse, tragic sentence: *"And he did not many mighty works there because of their unbelief"* (Matthew 13:58).

This teaches us that in the use of His miraculous power, Jesus requires faith, or a believing heart, in those who would be healed. He feels deep sorrow over the unbelief of the people He came to deliver.

One of the most thrilling questions Jesus ever asked is, *"Wilt thou be made whole?"* (John 5:6). His answer to a man who couldn't walk was, *"Rise, take up thy bed, and walk"* (v. 8). The Bible says what happened next: *"And immediately the man was made whole"* (v. 9). Faith does this.

God has the time and power and desire to save, to heal, to reward, and to bless. Wherever there is human need, He is present to heal (Luke 5:17).

God's desire and power to heal human life is still active today—in the faith and love of His people in all walks of life. God honors their faith, for their faith honors God.

Remember, one fact about faith is that Satan is the oppressor of human life, but God can bring life with health, peace, and happiness.

BELIEVE THE MESSAGE

It did not matter that the message for healing came to Naaman from a servant girl. The message of God is more important than the means by which it comes. We sometimes can lose sight of the importance of the message because of our insistence that the messenger carry our own label. But God does not compare people the way we do; He *"does not show favoritism"* (Romans 2:11 NIV). So when the apostle John complained to Jesus that the disciples saw someone casting out demons in Jesus's name even though he was not a follower, Jesus said, *"Do not forbid him, for no one who works a miracle in My name can soon afterward speak evil of Me. For he who is not against us is on our side"* (Mark 9:39–40 NKJV).

When the Holy Spirit led me to take His healing power to my generation, He had in mind a ministry that transcends denominational barriers. Our ministry is filled with God's love for *all people*. As long as we profess Jesus as our Savior, I believe that God asks us to love one another and work together to win souls.

GO WHERE THE POWER IS

Remember, the servant girl said, *"Would God my lord were with the prophet that is in Samaria! for he would recover him of his leprosy"* (2 Kings 5:3).

This is also the basis for the next way we use our faith for healing today.

Israel represented God; Elisha, who lived there, was God's prophet. In contrast, Syria was a land of idol worshipers, so Naaman had to get away from a sinful environment and get close to God. I believe the young girl, in essence, was telling him, "Go where the power is—back to God."

This is a profound truth—God is present everywhere at the same time because He is omnipresent, and He is omnipotent, having unlimited power and able to do anything. His all-prevailing power is available to us, but I believe it is important that we aim to maintain the right attitudes and faith that creates an atmosphere conducive to divine deliverance.

Even in His day, Christ found that some places were antagonistic to His truth, and He denounced these cities (Matthew 11:20–24).

General Naaman acted upon the advice of the young girl and set out on his trip ... but he made a serious mistake. Instead of going to the prophet, he went to see the king of Israel. King

Jehoram was outraged and declared he could do nothing for Naaman. About that time, a messenger came into the king's court with a word from Elisha: *"Let him come now to me, and he shall know that there is a prophet in Israel"* (2 Kings 5:8). This is important because it relates to the fourth way we can use our faith when we need healing.

PUT YOUR FAITH IN GOD, NOT PEOPLE

The girl had clearly said that the *prophet* would teach Naaman how to use his faith to be healed of leprosy. Instead, Naaman went to the king.

I cannot say it too much: I encourage you to put your faith in God. Have *confidence* in His servants or prophets, but put your *faith* in the Almighty, not another human being.

I believe the person God has chosen to help you receive healing is an instrument only—the means to an end—but that your deliverance comes by faith in God and His power.

Naaman rode to Elisha's house in his grand chariot. Having been forewarned by God that Naaman's attitude would need to be changed, and discerning the general's pride and arrogance, the prophet acted accordingly (2 Kings 5:9–10).

Elisha was a servant of God—the human instrument only. He was in the delicate position of having to deal with a proud, dying man and having to govern his actions according to the rules of faith. Faith had to be stirred up in Naaman; otherwise, he probably would have returned home with his leprosy. I have always believed that for the most part, to be healed, people's hearts should be right with God and their souls in tune with their Maker. There are many people God uses as instruments of healing, but I will always believe that the Healer is God.

In the Old Testament story of Naaman, Elisha remained in his house, detached from the general who had come to see him. He sent his servant to give the general a message: "*Go and wash in Jordan seven times, and thy flesh shall come again to thee, and thou shall be clean*" (2 Kings 5:10).

Naaman was astonished and then enraged at the prophet's instruction (2 Kings 5:11–12). As he walked away from the meeting with the messenger, I can imagine him saying, "Go dip in that filthy river? Bah! I thought the prophet would at least come to me and do some great thing and heal me. If I wanted to bathe, I would have stayed at home. At least the water in the rivers of Syria is clean."

Elisha saw him leave and perhaps thought, "Yes, that's the way it goes with the proud. They are bound by their own concepts and notions, never once thinking that when they ask for healing, they are dealing with Jehovah God and there are principles that govern faith." Humility, respect for God's message and His prophets, a desire to repent of sin and to worship the true God—these and other godly attitudes can help a person get in harmony with God and help him believe.

I believe many precious people are letting some preconceived idea or prejudice keep them from being healed. This thought may have occurred to one of Naaman's servants, who said, in my paraphrase of 2 Kings 5:13, "Master, we want our lord to be recovered from his leprosy. The prophet is right, Sir. You *were* expecting the prophet to do some great thing for you, and because he did the opposite, you were offended, and now you are returning unhealed. Master, in your servant's humble opinion, it is better to go wash and be clean."

What a wonderful way to reason things out.

ACCEPT GOD'S CORRECTION

Naaman listened, and when the servant finished speaking, I think he nodded his head in agreement. Perhaps in the language of his day, Naaman said something like, "You're right. I am wrong. I did come here self-centered and proud. Ah, this Elisha is a great one—saw right through me. And his God must have shown the prophet the kind of man I was. 'Go dip in the Jordan,' the prophet says. Sure. I can do that. Let's go."

I believe it takes a humble spirit for people to change their minds as remarkably as Naaman did. This is a marvelous thing. The Bible encourages us not to live for ourselves, but for Him (2 Corinthians 5:15). It says, *"If anyone is in Christ, he is a new creation; old things have passed away; behold, all things have become new"* (2 Corinthians 5:17 NKJV). I believe repentance starts with a change of mind before it becomes a change of heart.

With Elisha's message, *"Go and wash"* ringing in Naaman's ears, he plunged into the muddy, murky waters of the river Jordan. As he did so, 2 Kings 5:14 says, *"His flesh came again like unto the flesh of a little child, and he was clean."*

10

A POWERFUL STORY OF FAITH AND HEALING

In Mark 5:25–34 and Luke 8:43–48, we find the story of a woman who touched the hem of Jesus's garment and in return was healed and made whole. This biblical drama shows you how you can release your faith even under the most difficult conditions.

The name of the woman who touched the hem of Jesus's garment is unknown since it's not recorded in the Bible. I think this is because God would have us draw courage and inspiration from her story by putting our names where hers could have been. Then we, too, can release our faith, not by putting our hands on His clothes as she did, but by using some other point of contact that will enable us to believe Christ for our deliverance and receive from Him a healing just as glorious as she received.

SEVEN THINGS YOU CAN DO ON THE JOURNEY TOWARD HEALING

We can observe seven specific things the woman who touched the hem of Jesus's garment did on her journey toward healing, all of which we can also do.

1. She came to the end of her own way and stopped before her situation got the best of her.

The Bible says this woman had an incurable ailment—an issue of blood for twelve years. Something caused the bleeding that could not be cured. She *"had suffered many things of many physicians, and had spent all that she had, and was nothing bettered, but rather grew worse"* (Mark 5:26). She had spent every penny she had to regain her health, but her affliction grew steadily worse.

One day, she faced her problem and realized that she had exhausted her money as well as the medical knowledge of her day. This must have been a frustrating and perhaps even scary experience. She saw that all her efforts had been futile, and she made a remarkable decision—to stop before her situation got the best of her. She knew where she stood; she was beyond human help.

She came to the end of her own way and stopped.

2. She heard the story of faith—and believed it.

The woman with the issue of blood had heard about Jesus. She knew that a Galilean prophet was going throughout Judea, healing the sick and bringing peace to their souls. The Bible teaches that so remarkable was His power that lepers had been cleansed (Matthew 8:2–3; Mark 1:40–42; Luke 5:12–14); a paralytic had walked (Mark 2:1–12; Luke 5:17–26); a withered hand had been restored (Mark 3:1–5); and a centurion's servant had been healed (Luke 7:1–10). Naturally, great crowds were gathering around Jesus. The multitudes were so thick around Him that there was little opportunity to talk with Him or for Him to minister to people individually. But His ministry had inspired such faith that now people who even touched Him were healed. Luke 6:19 says, *"The whole multitude sought to touch him: for there went virtue out of him, and healed them all."*

The stories about Jesus were astounding, but the woman with the issue of blood must have believed them. Perhaps she realized that what a human being can do partially, God can do completely, and what mere mortals cannot do at all, our heavenly Father *can* do.

The story the woman heard about Jesus of Nazareth is the same one I heard when I had tuberculosis. I believed it, and through it, I found the way to faith and hope and was healed. This is the same story I've told throngs of people face-to-face in our evangelistic crusades and through the message on our radio and television programs.

I encourage you to believe this story of faith, for I believe that through it, you can do something about your frustrations, fears, and illnesses.

I would imagine this woman said to herself, "How wonderful this man must be! He heals those who just touch Him. That is the most amazing thing I have ever heard! They can reach out and touch Him, and He heals them. Think of that! If He can do it for them, He can do it for me. If they can touch Him, I can too. Oh, if I can touch just the hem of His robe, I know He will make me whole."

She knew that if she could just touch Jesus's clothes, her faith would be released.

3. She created a faith image of Jesus and of being healed by Him.

When the woman heard of Jesus and believed to the extent that she could set a point of contact for her faith, then Jesus's power became evident to her. He was no longer a name, a symbol, or a hope to others. He became a *Person* to her—One who could give her back her health and therefore her life. Her mind was filled with Him. I can only imagine that long before she saw Him, all other persons faded from her mind. The failures of the past faded away. All other ideas faded. All her other plans were laid aside so that her one plan was to make contact with Christ.

The Bible says, *"When she had heard of Jesus ... she said, If I may touch but his clothes, I shall be whole"* (Mark 5:27–28). It's like she saw Him in her mind before she saw Him with her eyes. I believe she saw herself there touching His clothes, feeling His healing power and being restored to health—before she ever moved toward Him.

I believe the woman's awareness of Jesus's healing power allowed her to move in faith, using Jesus's hem as a point of contact. Her faith and awareness of God's healing power put her mind in the right condition for healing. She knew the source of her healing was Jesus, and when she saw Him, she would believe and be made whole.

4. *She touched Jesus for a purpose.*

After the woman with the issue of blood had touched Jesus and felt that she had been healed, she *"declared unto him ... for what cause she had touched him, and how she was healed immediately"* (Luke 8:47).

Her cause was to be healed and made whole. For that purpose and with that goal in mind, she touched Him.

This woman pictured her whole self being made whole by touching Jesus's clothes. This was her cause, her dream, her goal. And this is why Jesus had come (1 John 3:8). He was within her reach when she went to touch Him.

5. *She used a point of contact to touch Him differently.*

The woman knew she needed to touch nothing more than Jesus's clothes (Mark 5:28). That was her point of contact.

There was no healing in His clothes, for He said to her, "*Thy faith hath made thee whole*" (Mark 5:34), *not* the touching of His clothes. It was her faith. But Jesus did not rebuke her for touching His clothes because she touched them as her point of contact with Him. She felt that by touching the robe He wore, she could believe.

I believe God will honor any biblical point of contact that helps us release our faith.

As the woman made her way through the crowd, I can almost hear her saying, "If I can only touch His clothes; if I can only touch His clothes!" I believe her faith cleared a path for her.

The day she went to see Jesus, the people were pressing so closely together that the only way she could have gotten through them was by faith. Faith can move God and people. It can take you through when everything else fails.

The woman pressed on through the people. And then— there He was! She had made it through to Him. She bent low, reached out a trembling hand, and *touched* the hem of His garment (Matthew 9:20). The mighty healing power of Christ was transferred from Him to her. It went all through her, into every fiber of her being, and released its force against her affliction. In a moment's time "*she felt in her body that she was healed of that plague*" (Mark 5:29). Notice, *she* was healed—not only her body, but her whole self.

Hundreds of people were around Christ and certainly touching Him. But this woman was the one there who touched the power of God in Him.

Oh, I pray you believe that Jesus is full of healing power! He is charged with the mighty power of God to make people whole in every way.

We do not read that anyone else in the crowd that day touched Jesus in the way the woman with the issue of blood reached out to Him. Hers was a different touch! She touched Him not as a part of the crowd but as an individual. She touched Him knowingly, believingly, purposefully, as a faith-filled point of contact. She touched His clothes with a specific purpose—to let her faith go to God. The moment she touched His robe, she demonstrated that she believed. Right then! This is the way I see a great demonstration of using a point of contact.

She said if she could touch Jesus's clothes, then and there she would believe that He would heal her. And it happened! I believe she would have been healed if she had used some other point of contact, so long as she had believed.

Something I believe we can take hold of is that there can be more than one way to use a point of contact because God is not limited to any special thing or to any certain person.

The simple purpose of a point of contact is to help us connect with the healing power of Jesus.

The apostle Paul sent handkerchiefs from his body, which he had prayed over, as points of contact to those who needed healing. The people knew Paul had prayed over the cloths and that there was power in his prayers. The moment the handkerchiefs were placed upon them—that moment, I believe—they sent their faith to God, and He healed them. Acts 19:11–12 says, *"And God wrought special miracles by the hands of Paul: so that from his body were brought unto the sick handkerchiefs or aprons, and the diseases departed from them, and the evil spirits went out of them."*

6. *She made contact with healing power.*

"She felt in her body that she was healed of that plague" (Mark 5:29). Contact was made between her faith and the healing power resident in Jesus Christ. Just as plugging a cord into an electrical outlet makes contact with the distant powerhouse, faith that is released—put into action—can make contact to release His healing power (James 2:20). This power, God's miraculous power, healed the woman of disease and made her whole.

7. *The faith she released made it possible for God's power to heal her.*

When Jesus asked, "Who touched my clothes?" the woman saw that she could not be hidden and came trembling before Him. She told Him why she had touched Him and how she had been healed.

Jesus said, *"Daughter, thy faith hath made thee whole; go in peace, and be whole of thy plague"* (Mark 5:34).

It seems as though the woman received from Jesus even more than she had hoped for. She had felt that her need was physical healing. But I believe He gave her what her whole inner being had been crying for—the shalom peace, with nothing missing and nothing broken, the kind of inner wholeness that only God and His Son can bring (Isaiah 26:3–4).

By connecting peace with healing, I like to think of Jesus saying, "You sought healing for your body. But healing is much more than just a physical work. Healing is also a spiritual work. Healing is wholeness and peace. Wholeness is healing for the spirit, soul, and body. Your faith has made *you* whole."

Jesus didn't just say that her faith made her physically well; He said it made her whole. Let us remember this: Healing from God is both physical and spiritual. Suppose the woman had received physical healing alone. She would have had healing for her body but perhaps not the peace of God in her soul. But when she looked to Jesus for her complete healing, she became centered in Him. When she touched His clothes, she was filled with His power and made whole.

What she did, I believe we can do. She sent her faith to God and so can you. God is a good God, and He rewards faith with deliverance and healing. Hebrew 11:6 (NIV) says, *"And without faith it is impossible to please God, because anyone who comes to him must believe that he exists and that he rewards those who earnestly seek him."*

PART 4

HEALING IS IN GOD'S HANDS

11

YOU CAN BE MADE WHOLE

In the healing of the paralyzed man described in Mark 2 and Luke 5, we see one of the New Testament's most remarkable examples of someone being made whole. Let's look at these passages together so we can refer to them throughout this chapter:

> And when he returned to Capernaum after some days, it was reported that he was at home. And many were gathered together, so that there was no more room, not even at the door. And he was preaching the word to them. And they came, bringing to him a paralytic carried by four men. And when they could not get near him because of the crowd, they removed the roof above him, and when they had made an opening, they let down the bed on which the paralytic lay. And when Jesus saw their faith, he said to the paralytic, "Son, your sins are forgiven." Now some of the scribes were sitting there, questioning in their hearts, "Why does this man speak

like that? He is blaspheming! Who can forgive sins but God alone?" And immediately Jesus, perceiving in his spirit that they thus questioned within themselves, said to them, "Why do you question these things in your hearts? Which is easier, to say to the paralytic, 'Your sins are forgiven,' or to say, 'Rise, take up your bed and walk'? But that you may know that the Son of Man has authority on earth to forgive sins"—he said to the paralytic—"I say to you, rise, pick up your bed, and go home." And he rose and immediately picked up his bed and went out before them all, so that they were all amazed and glorified God, saying, "We never saw anything like this!"

(Mark 2:1–12 ESV)

On one of those days, as he was teaching, Pharisees and teachers of the law were sitting there, who had come from every village of Galilee and Judea and from Jerusalem. And the power of the Lord was with him to heal. And behold, some men were bringing on a bed a man who was paralyzed, and they were seeking to bring him in and lay him before Jesus, but finding no way to bring him in, because of the crowd, they went up on the roof and let him down with his bed through the tiles into the midst before Jesus. And when he saw their faith, he said, "Man, your sins are forgiven you." And the scribes and the Pharisees began to question, saying, "Who is this who speaks blasphemies? Who can forgive sins but God alone?" When Jesus perceived their thoughts, he answered them, "Why do you question in your hearts? Which is easier, to say, 'Your sins are forgiven you,' or to say, 'Rise and walk'? But that you may know that the Son of Man has authority on earth to forgive sins"—he said to the man who was paralyzed—"I say to you, rise, pick up your bed and go home." And immediately he rose up before them and picked up what he had been lying on and went home, glorifying God. And amazement seized them all,

*and they glorified God and were filled with awe, saying, "We
have seen extraordinary things today." (Luke 5:17–26 ESV)*

Suffering with a severe case of paralysis, distant from the
interactions and activities of people who were well, this afflicted
man was a victim of the tormenting, enslaving power of the devil.
I have always believed and therefore preached that God did not
place this disease upon him, nor did God receive any glory from its
terrible effect upon his life and home.

Three things stand out in this man's deliverance: his great
physical need of healing; the presence of the Lord to heal him; and
the faith actions of his companions. The Bible says in Luke 5:17
that through Jesus, the Lord's power to heal was present when
someone is sick or afflicted.

God loves you, He is near to you, and He wants to heal you.
However, there is no magic connected with His divine healing. When I look at God's Word, I see that it's not about magic
power, but about faith in God's power. I believe active faith can
forge ahead in spite of every hindrance, every adversity—faith that
sometimes has to *raise the roof* to get the victory. And I've always
said, "Faith is where you find it."

Jesus came to bring life (John 10:10). He came not to afflict
but to heal (Matthew 19:2), not to destroy but to save (John 3:17),
not to impoverish but to enrich (2 Corinthians 9:11), not to bring
down but to lift up (Romans 15:13), not to send to hell but to
take to heaven (John 14:1–3). Jesus Christ came as a Healer, a
Deliverer, a Lifesaver.

Satan is a destroyer and oppressor. I pray you see that *"every
good gift and every perfect gift is from above, and cometh down from
the Father of lights, with whom is no variableness, neither shadow of
turning"* (James 1:17).

Jesus was always ready to heal the oppressed. Whenever the captives, who were believing by faith, could go where He was, they found deliverance. I encourage people to be careful not to separate any need we face from Christ's atoning work of Calvary. The teachings of Jesus are for a person's entire being—spirit, soul, and body. The Savior delivered those who came to Him in faith. In the same way, through the Holy Spirit, He can meet our needs today through His mighty healing power.

As Luke 5:17 declares, *"The power of the Lord was present to heal,"* and I believe that same power is available to heal today. Mark 16:18 declares, *"They shall lay hands on the sick, and they shall recover."* I see this as not only a privilege, but also a responsibility. As believers, we can honor this Scripture and lay hands on people when and where God directs and pray, believing for God to honor our faith and bring deliverance into the lives of those bound by the devil (Matthew 10:1; James 5:14–15).

James 5:16 says, *"Pray one for another, that ye may be healed."* We have the opportunity to pray for those suffering under the devil's oppression in a personal manner and pray for God to bring healing to one another.

FROM PARALYSIS TO FREEDOM

When Jesus was in Capernaum, the Bible says He was staying in a certain house that was crowded with people who had heard He was there. These people had come great distances to see and hear the mighty things of God. Even the Jewish leaders who opposed Jesus, the scribes and Pharisees, were present. So large was the crowd, there was not enough room for everybody, even around the door of the house (Mark 2:2).

Scripture tells us that the power of the Lord was present to heal the people in this crowd (Luke 5:17). This is God's provision for our deliverance from the oppression of the devil. Jesus was then, and is now, concerned with the needs of suffering humanity. He wants to set us free, and as Scripture says, our role in the process is to act in faith and believe in Him.

Four men in Capernaum had compassion on a paralyzed man and resolved to get him to Jesus for deliverance. I have always believed that compassion springs from divine love and is more than mere human sympathy. Compassion, to me, is an identification with people in their suffering until I feel like I *must* do something to get them into God's presence to see deliverance.

Having compassion for the paralytic man, these four men took his case into their own hands, taking him to Jesus, since he could not take himself to the healing service in Capernaum.

Before the four men took up the corners of the mattress on which the paralytic man lay, it seemed as though they pledged themselves to bold, direct action. They set out for their goal—deliverance.

Jesus had been in their city before, and His work of compassion to all who came for deliverance had most likely convinced them that He would turn away no one.

Confident that if they got their afflicted friend to the place where Jesus was, the man would return home whole in every way, they began moving toward Jesus, pressing through the crowd.

I believe this is the goal of an intercessor—to determine in your heart and mind that Christ must be reached. The idea is to know that you will reach Him as you press your way through. *"He that cometh to God must believe that He is, and that He is a rewarder of them that diligently seek him"* (Hebrews 11:6).

When they arrived with their friend, the four compassionate men found the way to Jesus was blocked by a crowd of people. As they advanced, seeking an opening, they were unsuccessful as the crowd was too thick. They kept trying, but each time, the human barrier stood in the way. Now what could they do? There was no opening in the crowd. It seemed that they had to return home defeated. But they refused to turn back; instead, they found a way to move forward.

We do not know how many times the four men tried to get their friend in to see Jesus. But I imagine there was one thing fixed in their minds: They would not turn back!

When all available means of getting to Jesus failed, these men of compassion threw caution to the wind so to speak and resorted to what seemed to be drastic action.

They raised the roof for victory.

These caring men faced a case of affliction beyond human cure. Only Jesus could heal their friend, but a human blockade stood between him and deliverance. Daring to go beyond the conventional, tossing pride aside, these men turned away from the crowd with what looked like a divinely conceived plan. With boldness, they climbed upon the housetop and began tearing off the roof. This kind of faith determination is the kind of crowd I want to be identified with—the roof raisers! Now, I'm not telling you to tear up someone's roof, but spiritually speaking, I believe it is time to spiritually raise the roof for our needs and get in where the Lord's power is present to heal.

These men were partners in their friend's deliverance. They felt they had a job to do—to get their suffering friend healed. The purpose of Jesus is to deliver humanity. We are His followers, and in some way as God directs, I believe we are all needed in God's kingdom to do something for the Lord.

God has promised victory to partners for deliverance. "Where two or three are gathered together in my name, there am I in the midst of them," Jesus said (Matthew 18:20). And remember that wherever the Lord is, His power is present to heal (Luke 5:17).

FAITH THAT WORKS

Imagine what the scene must have looked like. While Jesus was preaching to the people inside the house, there was a commotion on the housetop. These men were tearing off the tile roof!

I can imagine that as the debris filtered down into the house, the scribes and Pharisees murmured their disapproval. I wonder if they might have felt that such action was out of place because it interrupted the meeting.

Jesus was never alarmed by someone's faith for deliverance. He was there to *"preach the gospel to the poor ... to heal the brokenhearted, to preach deliverance to the captives, and recovering of sight to the blind, to set at liberty them that are bruised"* (Luke 4:18).

When an opportunity to deliver someone came, Jesus always went into action, setting the captive free. He preached to build faith, for *"faith cometh by hearing, and hearing by the word of God"* (Romans 10:17). When Jesus saw faith, He stopped whatever He was doing and responded.

Thank God, we are seeing this today.

My purpose in preaching and ministry is to inspire people to believe in God. I never want to be so tied to convention, to human plans, or to a set pattern that I will not stop—as God directs—to minister deliverance and healing to the souls and bodies of those in need.

In our story, as the Master looked up through the opening in the roof, He saw a makeshift bed being lowered by four pairs of strong hands. Then He saw something else, something that I believe He always looks for before He is moved into action. Luke 5:20 says, He *"saw their faith."*

Their faith was responsible for this scene. Their faith was set with the goal of deliverance and now, after tearing off the roof, they presented their friend in need to Christ the Healer.

BURNING BRIDGES

The compassionate faith partners had done all they could. Their faith had completed its mission. The roof was raised, an opening large enough to get their friend through to Jesus had been made. At last, the man afflicted by paralysis was where the power of the Lord was present to heal.

It was up to him now.

Jesus told the man in our story to get up, take up his bed, and go to his house (Luke 5:24). It was as though the time had come now for the paralytic to have personal faith, to set his goal, and to break every connection with the affliction, as he believed for deliverance. Others had told him of the Master. Others had brought him to the healing service, raised the roof for victory, and brought him before the healing presence of Christ. And now I believe it was his time to believe for his own miracle.

There is no magic connected with healing. The Bible shows that Jesus usually tells the unwell person, the captive, to do something; then He says, *"Thy faith hath made thee whole"* (Mark 5:34; 10:52; Luke 17:19). I have always thought that faith accomplishes things as it is *released or directed by God*. If you were to place a perfectly normal arm in a sling and keep it there in a state of inaction for several months, it could become difficult to move. Similarly, you might have faith lying dormant in your soul, but as you use it, as you exercise it, you can develop strength in that faith by hearing the Word of God. That's when I believe things can get moving spiritually.

The paralyzed man had been bedfast for a long time. By the outward appearance, his limbs were incapable of lifting and supporting his body. Spiritually speaking, it was like he had to sever all connections with past defeats and with present afflictions. His faith had to act. I believe Jesus was basically saying, "Arise!" to the man's inner person first. Then He said, "Take up your bed and walk." I see this as an example of how when the inner being stands up in faith, it can help the outer being take new strength into the body.

Without hesitation, the man recognized Jesus's authority over his affliction. And without questioning Christ's command of faith to rise up, take up his bed, and go home, he made an effort to rise. To the astonishment of the crowd, he actually *"rose up before them, and took up that whereon he lay, and departed to his own house, glorifying God"* (Luke 5:25).

I've always believed and therefore preached that there are no bonds that God cannot break, no fetters He cannot sever, no dungeon He cannot open, no disease He cannot heal, no victory He cannot win. Faith puts you directly into the hands of a limitless God who *"is able to do exceeding abundantly above all that we ask or think, according to the power that worketh in us"* (Ephesians 3:20).

If you are suffering today, I encourage you to believe *now.* There was a time when this man could have the miracle of healing working in his entire being and was that not the moment Jesus told him to rise?

I believe one of the main elements of healing is obedience to God and to His Word.

When the man arose under Jesus's healing power that went into his body, the crowd moved back to let him through. His destination now was home sweet home. He had been bound to his bed. But God, through faith in Him, had set him free.

As the people saw him go, they glorified God and said to each other, *"We have seen strange things to day"* (Luke 5:26). There is something about God's love and concern and healing for the captives bound by Satan's afflictions that can touch people's hearts and draw them toward God. The Bible says, *"The goodness of God leadeth thee to repentance"* (Romans 2:4).

RAISE THE ROOF FOR VICTORY—FOR YOURSELF AND OTHERS!

I believe we must have revivals to bring healing to the whole person. The power of God must fall upon us. The power of the Lord must be present for our deliverance. The hurts and ills of humanity can find deliverance through our prayers of faith.

Dare we fail God and suffering people in this crucial hour of the world's need? Shall we sit idly by while Satan is busy in his work of human oppression, when the kind of revival conducted by Jesus, the disciples, and missionaries of the early church was to heal people in spirit, soul, and body? Why not now? Why not raise the roof for victory?

The same Christ who healed the paralyzed man's afflictions also said to him, *"Thy sins are forgiven thee"* (Luke 5:20).

The man went home saved and healed. He was *whole*.

I encourage you to place yourself in an atmosphere like this man who found healing. Ask God how you can spiritually raise the roof for victory! I believe healing today is available by faith in the same Christ who healed the paralyzed man and who lives today to meet your every need for health, healing, and wholeness.

GOD'S HEALING POWER

I believe the Lord's healing for our bodies and lives is one of the truly magnificent proofs of His personal concern for everything that affects us. His healing power stands out to me as one of the great love forces of all time. I see it as the outstretched hand of God. His thoughts are revealed in miraculous action toward you and me. Perhaps it's because I had such a personal need for healing that I love the healing power of Jesus Christ and believe humanity will always need His healing touch!

The great healing power of Jesus Christ can be readily available to us. We can't see it any more than we can see the wind. We can *hear* the wind and *feel* the wind, but we cannot see it. This is much like the Spirit of God and His healing power. We can feel the great healing power of God and experience it, but in my case, I cannot really *explain* its tangibility to anyone.

Many people want me to explain my ministry of healing, to tell them why I pray for the sick, and they ask, "How can this particular disease be healed by prayer?"

Well, in the first place, there are many different godly delivery systems for healing. I believe all of them, even those that are more natural than supernatural, are ultimately given to us by God in His truly great love for us all.

So, here are the things I've learned that I can do when I am in need, and I pray these give you some insight as to what you can do to make this more personal to you:

1. PRAY

The Bible says, "*Let him pray*" (James 5:13). When you're in need, the Bible says you should pray. During that time, the study of the Bible can be an insightful addition to prayer. When I have suffered in any way, I inevitably wind up reading my Bible. I often take it to bed with me. Sometimes I have it very near me while I try to sleep. I have enormous confidence in the results of reading my Bible, searching the Scriptures, and reading certain passages out loud to myself. I have sometimes read a specific passage, such as Psalm 23, as many as five times aloud to myself. If James were with us today, I believe he might say, "Let him pray. Let him read his

Bible. Let him contemplate God and his own life. Let him think about his whole self and let him meditate."

2. CALL FOR HELP

The Bible offers us this valuable step: *"Let him call for the elders"* (James 5:14). In other words, let him call for the spiritual leaders of the church. As believers, the church is central in our lives. It is the body of Christ, and I believe the person who ignores Christ's church is ignoring the great fundamental healing force in our world today.

Why do I emphasize the calling so much? Because I have discovered the enormous ability of believers in the church to believe for healing. I have found the act of calling for prayer is an act of faith. It helps me release my faith. It becomes, in effect, a *point of contact* for the releasing of faith.

"Let him call for the elders [spiritual leaders] *of the church; and let them pray over him ... the **prayer of faith"*** (James 5:14–15).

12

ULTIMATE HEALING

I believe Christ our Lord has one other healing instrument, the most powerful one and the ultimate cure.

What is it? The resurrection, the ultimate healing of your total being. *The resurrection!*

THE END OF EARTHLY LIFE ISN'T THE END

I thrill at every healing act of God. To me, all healing is divine—your salvation by faith in the death and resurrection of Jesus Christ. I believe your deliverance from fear, frustration, and inner conflicts; the supplying of your financial needs; your body getting well or even better; your sense of great well-being; your entrance into miracle-living; your guidance into a career that is right for you; your use of prayer—all of these and more can be part of God's healing power for you. I believe cooperating with the life forces God has put here for us can contribute to our better health and miracle-living.

My prayer for every human being is that once their appointed time on earth has finished, their acceptance of Jesus Christ as their Savior and Lord will usher them into heaven for their ultimate miracle: the reward of eternal life with Him.

A CONVERSATION WITH A YOUNG COUPLE

There is a young couple, parents of three small children, who are very close to me in helping bring people into a greater faith for better health and miracle-living. They said to me, "We have seen many healings, even things we believe are miracles. Still, people die, don't they?"

Before I could reply, the young wife said, "You know, death is something we don't talk about; we don't seem to realize there is death. We are so young, we don't encounter death often. But everybody should realize that at some point after our earthly journey is up, we are going to die."

I said, "One thing we must keep foremost in our thinking and believing is the resurrection."

The husband said, "Yes, we believe in the resurrection but how does that relate to the healing of sickness?"

I said, "It relates in every way because whatever medical science, prayer, or any other healing instrument misses, the resurrection will get!"

"That's wonderful," he said. "But how?"

I responded, "Because the resurrection is about a Person, the Person of our Savior and Lord, Jesus Christ, who told us in John 11:25 that He is *'the resurrection, and the life.'* The resurrection is not a thing; it is our risen Lord waiting to give us the fullness of life, to restore everything which has diminished us on earth, including our bodies, in any way. It's complete healing, it's immortality, it's whole-person life made eternal, it's life after death in the same way that Christ lives in His glorified body."

My young friends almost shouted when they cried out, "Super! Super!"

Turning to each other, they said, "I'm glad I'm a Christian, aren't you?"

For me, being a Christian is the greatest thing in the world. We serve a risen Savior who says in John 14:1–3, *"Let not your heart be troubled: ye believe in God, believe also in me. In my Father's house are many mansions: if it were not so, I would have told you. I go to prepare a place for you. And if I go and prepare a place for you, I will come again, and receive you unto myself; that where I am, there ye may be also."* And in John 14:19, Jesus says, *"Because I live, ye shall live also."*

THIS IS WHAT I BELIEVE SUSTAINED PAUL

I believe the Bible with all my being. To me, it is the Word of God, and it speaks God's life to me daily. It's also the explanation of life here and after death, and what to do about it. It is the only Book that does that for me.

Paul, who wrote so much of our New Testament, really opens up the healing and restorative powers that come through the resurrection. It sustained him when he was:

+ Stoned and left for dead (Acts 14:19–20)

+ Held in filthy prisons in Philippi (Acts 16:23–24), Caesarea (Acts 24:27), and Rome (Acts 28:30)

+ Shipwrecked several times (Acts 27:39–44; 2 Corinthians 11:25)

+ Beaten and scarred (2 Corinthians 11:24–25)

+ Persecuted until he despaired of his life (2 Corinthians 11:26)

+ Hit with weariness and pain (2 Corinthians 11:27)

+ Hungry and thirsty (Philippians 4:12)

+ Cold and without proper clothes for warmth (2 Corinthians 11:27)

+ Satan's messenger struck him with a thorn in his flesh (2 Corinthians 12:7)

+ He was forsaken by his closest friends (2 Timothy 4:10)

+ He labored so hard that no one equaled him (1 Corinthians 15:10)

+ His prayers were not always granted or answered the way he asked (2 Corinthians 12:8–10)

When Paul was dealing with what could have been fear within himself and others and deadly negative forces warred against him, I believe he was also sustained by the hope he found in the gospel as well as the prayers and care of the early church. But to him, it seems, the most important thing was knowing Jesus *"and the power of his resurrection"* (Philippians 3:10). I believe this is the greatest hope for you and me too.

ENCOURAGEMENT FROM THE LIFE OF PAUL

I like Paul very much because he faced many situations I relate to, and in some ways, perhaps you can relate to them as well. Let's look at some of Paul's beliefs, beliefs that may help you as you walk with God in wholeness.

1. *He believed he could bear whatever happened to him as long as he knew he had God's grace.*

When the satanic messenger bore in on his flesh with opposition, metaphorically like a thorn sticking into his body, he prayed three times for God to remove it. When God did not do so, Paul stood up to it until God spoke in his heart: *"My grace is sufficient for thee: for my strength is made perfect in weakness"* (2 Corinthians 12:9).

It was then that Paul knew God's grace was strong enough to see him through even the thorny messenger of Satan and he could relax, knowing he could win. He knew then that nothing could defeat his spirit. Nothing could break his hold on his faith in God, or God's in him. Nothing earthly or from the enemy could put him down and keep him down. Such is the power we can find in knowing that we have God's grace in our hearts and our lives.

The way I encourage myself when I feel the need is to remember that God is all-powerful. God is in me, and I am in Him. His grace is real in my life. I am not alone. *God is with me. ME.* I get very personal about it. The grace of God that I feel in my heart is the overall sustaining power that has kept me steady and kept me going with a good attitude and positive faith. His grace makes me know God loves me, God believes in me, and God is with me. In my weakness and even my mistakes, He becomes more real to me as we walk together.

2. Paul practiced seed-faith living.

Paul urges us to remember the words of the Lord Jesus, reminding us how He said, *"It is more blessed to give than to receive"* (Acts 20:35).

I believe it is blessed to give and also important to recognize that Scripture tells us that what one gives is multiplied back. Jesus said in Luke 6:38, *"Give, and it shall be given unto you; good measure, pressed down, and shaken together, and running over."*

It is Paul who said of the Lord, *"God loveth a cheerful giver"* (2 Corinthians 9:7). For me, it's wanting to give until I just can't wait to do it.

It is Paul who takes us back to God's eternal law of sowing and reaping from Genesis 8:22, where the Creator said, *"While the earth remaineth, seedtime and harvest ... shall not cease."*

I refer to this as the eternal seed-faith principle upon which a person's successful scriptural obedience to seed-faith living is based. Sowing, then reaping, is a matter of biblical life. Paul said of this eternal law of God, *"He which soweth sparingly shall reap also sparingly; and he which soweth bountifully shall reap also bountifully"* (2 Corinthians 9:6).

Notice, Paul refers to *"He which soweth..."* This is where we can be the sowers. Then as a result, we also can be the ones who reap. And we can sow *or* reap either sparingly or bountifully. Sparing or scanty sowing produces a scanty harvest. Bountiful sowing produces a full harvest.

It is Paul who said every man is to give with purpose in his heart—in essence, starting with his spirit, his inner self—not grudgingly or of necessity but giving because there is a purpose for it (2 Corinthians 9:7).

Paul also said if you give and don't do so with love, your giving will profit you nothing; you are like someone throwing something infinitely valuable away (1 Corinthians 13:3).

The Gospel of Luke says if you give with love, *"your reward shall be great"* (Luke 6:35).

Paul spoke of giving *and* receiving as being inextricably woven together, inseparably linked, working together to create a godly wholeness. He told the church at Philippi, *"No church communicated with me as concerning giving and receiving, but ye only. ... Not because I desire a gift: but I desire fruit* [or harvest] *that may abound to your account"* (Philippians 4:15, 17).

Paul said givers have an account with God that they can draw on. You give first and God has designed it so that you will receive, just as day follows night (Genesis 8:22). After you breathe out, you breathe in. In the same way, after you give, you can receive.

Paul follows up his explanation of giving and receiving by saying, *"But my God **shall supply all your need** according to his riches in glory by Christ Jesus"* (Philippians 4:19).

No other New Testament writer used such strong, unequivocable words. Why? I believe it was because Paul had such tough experiences that he had to learn the way into God's rich grace and God's sure way of giving back to him so he could sustain his life abundantly to the very end.

I believe this with my whole being. I practice giving cheerfully and giving first. I practice making God the Source of my total supply. I expect to receive from my giving; I expect a miracle, many miracles, miracle-living.

I got it from the Bible, but especially through Paul as he got it from Jesus.

Paul's seed-faith living gave him God's strength made perfect. By planting the seed first, he uprooted the weeds such as hate, envy, jealousy, malice, bitterness, and every kind of deadly thing that came against him.

I believe Paul planted the seed of love when he was hated, the seed of respect when disrespected, the seed of giving when no one gave to him, and the seed of approval when disapproved.

He gave concern, care, and compassion; he prayed for others' healing. The grace of God and the power of Christ made him strong (2 Corinthians 12:9). Paul was attacked so viciously that he was left for dead, but he said, "*For Christ's sake, I delight in weaknesses, in insults, in hardships, in persecutions, in difficulties. For when I am weak, then I am strong*" (2 Corinthians 12:10 NIV).

Paul was able to rise up, face life at its meanest and death at its bitterest, and say: "*I have fought a good fight, I have finished my course, I have kept the faith: Henceforth there is laid up for me a crown of righteousness, which the Lord ... shall give me at that day: and not to me only*" (2 Timothy 4:7–8).

Once he became a servant of God, Paul waged a good fight, and it appeared as if there was no hate, bitterness, envy, or murder in his heart. And when the fight was over, he was still ready to enter into heaven.

3. Paul kept his faith in God.

For Paul to have kept his faith in God is a miracle for the days in which he lived, as it is in our time. Every corruption we face is similar to the rampant corruption in Paul's path. The devil was as much the devil then as he is now, so was the messenger he sent to harass and hurt Paul. People attacked Paul and left him for dead. But the Christ living in him, in the unlimited power of the Holy Spirit, could not be shaken or left for dead. Christ standing up in Paul gave His strength to him so that Paul was also able to stand up, his faith intact, his belief strong and unabated, his inner knowing as strong as heaven itself.

4. Paul finished his course.

God set Paul on a course, just as I think God has a course for your life and for mine.

That course was to serve God, to share Christ with others, and to plant seeds of His love in people's lives in good times and bad times, when it was easy and when it was hard. And Paul did it! What a great thing to realize: Paul finished his course.

THE RESURRECTION

Always ahead of Paul was the fact of the resurrection. It beckoned him on. He knew that Jesus had given His life on the cross as the Son of God and was also *"the seed of David"* (2 Timothy 2:8). As a seed, He was planted for all people. Paul knew that seed burst into harvest, and that harvest was the greatest miracle of all—the resurrection. First, the resurrection of *the seed of the woman* promised by God in Genesis 3:15 and the resurrection of Jesus's own life as a seed.

Paul knew that the hope of that resurrection was his too—as well as mine, yours, and all those who live in Christ Jesus.

It was the fact of the resurrection shining like the noonday sun before Paul that made death palatable to him, that took away its sting, making it a grand passage from this earthly life to the heavenly life where there is no more sickness, no more pain, no more lack, no more tears, and no more death (Revelation 7:16–17).

The seeds I am planting are not for nothing. Already, every day, God is multiplying them back and my life is counting for Him. Every seed multiplied helps to replenish my spirit. It helps my body, my finances, my soul, and my spirit. It's a direct and personal forerunner of the resurrection I shall have.

I have a good fight to engage in.

I have God's faith in my heart to keep intact and active.

I have a course, God's plan for my life, to complete, little by little, day by day.

I have a crown laid up for me; it's there waiting.

I believe that Christ makes all of our lives worthwhile—both here on earth and in the resurrection. First Corinthians 15:54 (NIV) says, *"When the perishable has been clothed with the imperishable, and the mortal with immortality, then the saying that is written will come true: 'Death has been swallowed up in victory.'"* (See Isaiah 25:8.) This ascent to heaven after life as a believer in Jesus can be the greatest victory we have ever known.

AFFIRM YOUR FAITH IN THE RESURRECTION

Now that you have read this chapter and are coming to understand how powerful the resurrection is, you can say to yourself with total confidence:

+ The ultimate healing of my total being is the resurrection.

+ I believe that like Paul, whatever happens to me, I can expect a miracle. I can do what I'm called to do so long as I know I have God's grace in my life.

+ I believe, like Paul, that sowing and reaping is a matter of life itself. If I sow sparingly, I will reap sparingly—but if I sow bountifully, I shall reap bountifully. So I will plant many good seeds in this life.

+ Like Paul, I will keep my faith in God and finish my course, knowing there is a crown laid up for me and death will be swallowed up in victory.

APPENDIX:
SCRIPTURES ON HEALING AND FAITH

I believe God is a good God who wants to heal you. As you apply these healing Scriptures to your life, release your faith and be healed in Jesus's name.

I am the LORD that healeth thee. (Exodus 15:26)

And ye shall serve the LORD your God, and he shall bless thy bread, and thy water; and I will take sickness away from the midst of thee. (Exodus 23:25)

It came to pass after these things, that the son of the woman, the mistress of the house, fell sick; and his sickness was so sore, that there was no breath left in him. ... And he [Elijah] stretched himself upon the child three times, and cried unto the Lord, *and said, O* Lord *my God, I pray thee, let this child's soul come into him again. And the* Lord *heard the voice of Elijah; and the soul of the child came into him again, and he revived.* (1 Kings 17:17, 21–22)

Naaman, captain of the host of the king of Syria ... was a leper. ... So Naaman came with his horses and with his chariot, and stood at the door of the house of Elisha. And Elisha sent a messenger unto him, saying, Go and wash in Jordan seven times, and thy flesh shall come again to thee, and thou shalt be clean. ... Then went he down, and dipped himself seven times in Jordan, according to the saying of the man of God: and his flesh came again like unto the flesh of a little child, and he was clean. (2 Kings 5:1, 9–10, 14)

O Lord *my God, I cried unto thee, and thou hast healed me.* (Psalm 30:2)

Bless the Lord, *O my soul: and all that is within me, bless his holy name. Bless the* Lord, *O my soul, and forget not all his benefits: who forgiveth all thine iniquities; who healeth all thy diseases; who redeemeth thy life from destruction; who crowneth thee with lovingkindness and tender mercies; who satisfieth thy mouth with good things; so that thy youth is renewed like the eagle's.* (Psalm 103:1–5)

He sent his word, and healed them, and delivered them from their destructions.   (Psalm 107:20)

He healeth the broken in heart, and bindeth up their wounds.   (Psalm 147:3)

My son, attend to my words; incline thine ear unto my sayings. Let them not depart from thine eyes; keep them in the midst of thine heart. For they are life unto those that find them, and health to all their flesh. Keep thy heart with all diligence; for out of it are the issues of life.   (Proverbs 4:20–23)

In those days was Hezekiah sick unto death. And Isaiah the prophet the son of Amoz came unto him, and said unto him, Thus saith the LORD, Set thine house in order: for thou shalt die, and not live. Then Hezekiah turned his face toward the wall, and prayed unto the LORD, and said, Remember now, O LORD, I beseech thee, how I have walked before thee in truth and with a perfect heart, and have done that which is good in thy sight. And Hezekiah wept sore. Then came the word of the LORD to Isaiah, saying, Go, and say to Hezekiah, Thus saith the LORD, the God of David thy father, I have heard thy prayer, I have seen thy tears: behold, I will add unto thy days fifteen years.   (Isaiah 38:1–5)

The writing of Hezekiah king of Judah, when he had been sick, and was recovered of his sickness: … The living, the living, he shall praise thee, as I do this day: the father to the children shall make known thy truth.   (Isaiah 38:9, 19)

They that wait upon the LORD *shall renew their strength; they shall mount up with wings as eagles; they shall run, and not be weary; and they shall walk, and not faint.*   (Isaiah 40:31)

Surely he hath borne our griefs, and carried our sorrows: yet we did esteem him stricken, smitten of God, and afflicted. But he was wounded for our transgressions, he was bruised for our iniquities: the chastisement of our peace was upon him; and with his stripes we are healed.   (Isaiah 53:4–5)

For I will restore health unto thee, and I will heal thee of thy wounds, saith the LORD.   (Jeremiah 30:17)

But unto you that fear my name shall the Sun of righteousness arise with healing in his wings.   (Malachi 4:2)

Jesus went about all Galilee, teaching in their synagogues, and preaching the gospel of the kingdom, and healing all manner of sickness and all manner of disease among the people.
(Matthew 4:23)

When Jesus was entered into Capernaum, there came unto him a centurion, beseeching him, and saying, Lord, my servant lieth at home sick of the palsy, grievously tormented. And Jesus saith unto him, I will come and heal him. The centurion answered and said, Lord, I am not worthy that thou shouldest come under my roof: but speak the word only, and my servant shall be healed. For I am a man under authority, having soldiers under me: and I say to this man, Go, and he goeth; and to another, Come, and he cometh; and to my servant, Do this, and he doeth it. When Jesus heard it, he marvelled, and said to them that followed, Verily I say unto you, I have not found so great faith, no, not in Israel. ... And Jesus said unto the centurion, Go thy way; and as thou hast believed, so be it done unto thee. And his servant was healed in the selfsame hour.
(Matthew 8:5–10, 13)

They brought unto him many that were possessed with devils: and he cast out the spirits with his word, and healed all that were sick: that it might be fulfilled which was spoken by Esaias [Isaiah] the prophet, saying, Himself took our infirmities, and bare our sicknesses. (Matthew 8:16–17)

When he had called unto him his twelve disciples, he gave them power against unclean spirits, to cast them out, and to heal all manner of sickness and all manner of disease.
(Matthew 10:1)

Then Jesus answered and said unto her, O woman, great is thy faith: be it unto thee even as thou wilt. And her daughter was made whole from that very hour. (Matthew 15:28)

Great multitudes came unto him, having with them those that were lame, blind, dumb, maimed, and many others, and cast them down at Jesus' feet; and he healed them: insomuch that the multitude wondered, when they saw the dumb to speak, the maimed to be whole, the lame to walk, and the blind to see: and they glorified the God of Israel.   (Matthew 15:30–31)

Two blind men sitting by the way side, when they heard that Jesus passed by, cried out, saying, Have mercy on us, O Lord, thou son of David. And the multitude rebuked them, because they should hold their peace: but they cried the more, saying, Have mercy on us, O Lord, thou son of David. And Jesus stood still, and called them, and said, What will ye that I shall do unto you? They say unto him, Lord, that our eyes may be opened. So Jesus had compassion on them, and touched their eyes: and immediately their eyes received sight, and they followed him.   (Matthew 20:30–34)

The blind and the lame came to him in the temple; and he healed them.   (Matthew 21:14)

For he had healed many; insomuch that they pressed upon him for to touch him, as many as had plagues. And unclean spirits, when they saw him, fell down before him, and cried, saying, Thou art the Son of God.   (Mark 3:10–11)

He ordained twelve, that they should be with him, and that he might send them forth to preach, and to have power to heal sicknesses, and to cast out devils.   (Mark 3:14–15)

One of the multitude answered and said, Master, I have brought unto thee my son, which hath a dumb spirit; and wheresoever he taketh him, he teareth him: and he foameth, and gnasheth with his teeth, and pineth away. … If thou canst do any thing, have compassion on us, and help us. Jesus said unto him, If thou canst believe, all things are possible to him that believeth. And straightway the father of the child cried out, and said with tears, Lord, I believe; help thou mine unbelief. When Jesus saw that the people came running together, he rebuked the foul spirit, saying unto him, Thou dumb and deaf spirit, I charge thee, come out of him, and enter no more into him. And the spirit cried, and rent him sore, and came out of him: and he was as one dead; insomuch that many said, He is dead. But Jesus took him by the hand, and lifted him up; and he arose. (Mark 9:17–18, 22–27)

And these signs shall follow them that believe; In my name shall they cast out devils; they shall speak with new tongues; they shall take up serpents; and if they drink any deadly thing, it shall not hurt them; they shall lay hands on the sick, and they shall recover. (Mark 16:17–18)

The Spirit of the Lord is upon me, because he hath anointed me to preach the gospel to the poor; he hath sent me to heal the brokenhearted, to preach deliverance to the captives, and recovering of sight to the blind, to set at liberty them that are bruised. (Luke 4:18)

It came to pass on a certain day, as he was teaching, that there were Pharisees and doctors of the law sitting by, which were come out of every town of Galilee, and Judaea, and Jerusalem: and the power of the Lord was present to heal them. And, behold, men brought in a bed a man which was taken with a palsy: and they sought means to bring him in, and to lay him before him. And when they could not find by what way they might bring him in because of the multitude, they went upon the housetop, and let him down through the tiling with his couch into the midst before Jesus. And when he saw their faith, he said unto him, Man, thy sins are forgiven thee. And the scribes and the Pharisees began to reason, saying, Who is this which speaketh blasphemies? Who can forgive sins, but God alone? But when Jesus perceived their thoughts, he answering said unto them, What reason ye in your hearts? Whether is easier, to say, Thy sins be forgiven thee; or to say, Rise up and walk? But that ye may know that the Son of man hath power upon earth to forgive sins, (he said unto the sick of the palsy,) I say unto thee, Arise, and take up thy couch, and go into thine house. And immediately he rose up before them, and took up that whereon he lay, and departed to his own house, glorifying God. (Luke 5:17–25)

The whole multitude sought to touch him: for there went virtue out of him, and healed them all. (Luke 6:19)

In that same hour he cured many of their infirmities and plagues, and of evil spirits; and unto many that were blind he gave sight. Then Jesus answering said unto them, Go your way, and tell John what things ye have seen and heard; how that the blind see, the lame walk, the lepers are cleansed, the deaf hear, the dead are raised, to the poor the gospel is preached.

(Luke 7:21–22)

A woman having an issue of blood twelve years, which had spent all her living upon physicians, neither could be healed of any, came behind him, and touched the border of his garment: and immediately her issue of blood stanched. And Jesus said, Who touched me? When all denied, Peter and they that were with him said, Master, the multitude throng thee and press thee, and sayest thou, Who touched me? And Jesus said, Somebody hath touched me: for I perceive that virtue is gone out of me. And when the woman saw that she was not hid, she came trembling, and falling down before him, she declared unto him before all the people for what cause she had touched him, and how she was healed immediately. And he said unto her, Daughter, be of good comfort: thy faith hath made thee whole; go in peace. (Luke 8:43–48)

Then he called his twelve disciples together, and gave them power and authority over all devils, and to cure diseases. And he sent them to preach the kingdom of God, and to heal the sick. (Luke 9:1–2)

Heal the sick … and say unto them, The kingdom of God is come nigh unto you. (Luke 10:9)

There was a woman which had a spirit of infirmity eighteen years, and was bowed together, and could in no wise lift up herself. And when Jesus saw her, he called her to him, and said unto her, Woman, thou art loosed from thine infirmity. And he laid his hands on her: and immediately she was made straight, and glorified God. (Luke 13:11–13)

Jesus saith unto him, Rise, take up thy bed, and walk. And immediately the man was made whole, and took up his bed, and walked. (John 5:8–9)

Then they took away the stone from the place where the dead was laid. And Jesus lifted up his eyes, and said, Father, I thank thee that thou hast heard me. And I knew that thou hearest me always: but because of the people which stand by I said it, that they may believe that thou hast sent me. And when he thus had spoken, he cried with a loud voice, Lazarus, come forth. And he that was dead came forth, bound hand and foot with graveclothes: and his face was bound about with a napkin. Jesus saith unto them, Loose him, and let him go. (John 11:41–44)

Peter and John went up together into the temple at the hour of prayer, being the ninth hour. And a certain man lame from his mother's womb was carried, whom they laid daily at the gate of the temple which is called Beautiful, to ask alms of them that entered into the temple; who seeing Peter and John about to go into the temple asked an alms. And Peter, fastening his eyes upon him with John, said, Look on us. And he gave heed unto them, expecting to receive something of them. Then Peter said, Silver and gold have I none; but such as I have give I thee: In the name of Jesus Christ of Nazareth rise up and walk. And he took him by the right hand, and lifted him up: and immediately his feet and ankle bones received strength. And he leaping up stood, and walked, and entered with them into the temple, walking, and leaping, and praising God. And all the people saw him walking and praising God: and they knew that it was he which sat for alms at the Beautiful gate of the temple: and they were filled with wonder and amazement at that which had happened unto him. (Acts 3:1–10)

There came also a multitude out of the cities round about unto Jerusalem, bringing sick folks, and them which were vexed with unclean spirits: and they were healed every one.
(Acts 5:16)

There sat a certain man at Lystra, impotent in his feet, being a cripple from his mother's womb, who never had walked: the same heard Paul speak: who stedfastly beholding him, and perceiving that he had faith to be healed, said with a loud voice, Stand upright on thy feet. And he leaped and walked.
(Acts 14:8–10)

It came to pass, that the father of Publius lay sick of a fever and of a bloody flux: to whom Paul entered in, and prayed, and laid his hands on him, and healed him. So when this was done, others also, which had diseases in the island, came, and were healed. (Acts 28:8–9)

Let us therefore come boldly unto the throne of grace, that we may obtain mercy, and find grace to help in time of need. (Hebrews 4:16)

Lift up the hands which hang down, and the feeble knees; and make straight paths for your feet, lest that which is lame be turned out of the way; but let it rather be healed. (Hebrews 12:12–13)

Is any sick among you? let him call for the elders of the church; and let them pray over him, anointing him with oil in the name of the Lord: and the prayer of faith shall save the sick, and the Lord shall raise him up; and if he have committed sins, they shall be forgiven him. Confess your faults one to another, and pray one for another, that ye may be healed. The effectual fervent prayer of a righteous man availeth much. (James 5:14–16)

Who his own self bare our sins in his own body on the tree, that we, being dead to sins, should live unto righteousness: by whose stripes ye were healed. (1 Peter 2:24)

Beloved, I wish above all things that thou mayest prosper and be in health, even as thy soul prospereth.　　　(3 John 1:2)

He shewed me a pure river of water of life, clear as crystal, proceeding out of the throne of God and of the Lamb. In the midst of the street of it, and on either side of the river, was there the tree of life, which bare twelve manner of fruits, and yielded her fruit every month: and the leaves of the tree were for the healing of the nations.　　　(Revelation 22:1–2)

ABOUT THE AUTHOR

Granville Oral Roberts (1918–2009) was one of the most influential Christian leaders of the twentieth century.

At age seventeen, Oral was healed of tuberculosis at a tent revival meeting. In 1947, he established the Oral Roberts Evangelistic Association in Tulsa, Oklahoma. Throughout his ministry, he conducted more than three hundred healing crusades in over thirty-five countries across six continents.

In 1955, Oral began televising the healing crusades, bringing evangelism into living rooms across America. This sparked his weekly healing television programs and several prime-time specials.

Three years later, Oral established the Abundant Life Prayer Group, which has received over 29 million phone calls for prayer to date.

In 1963, he founded Oral Roberts University in Tulsa, Oklahoma, with the goal of developing whole-person leaders empowered by the Holy Spirit. In 1981, he established the City of Faith Medical and Research Center, with the mission of merging medicine and prayer as God had revealed it to him.

Oral was married to "his darling wife," Evelyn Lutman Roberts, for more than sixty-six years. He wrote over 130 books, including *The Miracle of Seed Faith* and his autobiography, *Expect a Miracle*, as well as many other inspirational materials.

This book includes excerpts from Oral's book *If You Need Healing Do These Things* as well as some of his other writings on healing and miracles. *Oral Roberts on Healing: Living in God's Miracles* was compiled by his son and daughter-in-law, Richard and Lindsay Roberts, who spread the good news of Jesus worldwide through Richard Roberts Ministries.

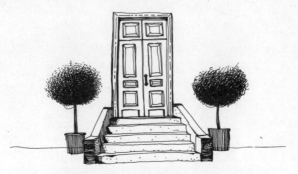

Welcome to Our House!

We Have a Special Gift for You

It is our privilege and pleasure to share in your love of Christian books. We are committed to bringing you authors and books that feed, challenge, and enrich your faith.

To show our appreciation, we invite you to sign up to receive a specially selected **Reader Appreciation Gift**, with our compliments. Just go to the Web address at the bottom of this page.

God bless you as you seek a deeper walk with Him!

WE HAVE A GIFT FOR YOU. VISIT:

whpub.me/nonfictionthx

WHITAKER
HOUSE